WORKBOOK TO ACCOMPANY INTRODUCTION TO BIOSTATISTICAL APPLICATIONS IN HEALTH RESEARCH WITH MICROSOFT® OFFICE EXCEL®

ROBERT P. HIRSCH
Foundation for the Advanced Education in the Sciences

WILEY

Published by John Wiley & Sons, Inc., Hoboken, New Jersey
Published simultaneously in Canada

For general information on our other products and services or for technical support, please contact our Customer Care Department within the United States at (800) 762–2974, outside the United States at (317) 572–3993 or fax (317) 572–4002.

Wiley also publishes its books in a variety of electronic formats. Some content that appears in print may not be available in electronic formats. For more information about Wiley products, visit our web site at www.wiley.com.

Library of Congress Cataloging-in-Publication Data:

Name: Hirsch, Robert P., author.
Title: Introduction to biostatistical applications in health research with Microsoft Office Excel / Robert P. Hirsch.
Description: New York, NY : John Wiley & Sons Inc., 2016.
Identifiers: LCCN 2015039977 | ISBN: 9781119089650 (cloth) | ISBN: 9781119089865 (workbook)
Subjects: | MESH: Microsoft Excel (Computer file) | Biostatistics–methods. | Data Interpretation, Statistical. | Mathematical Computing.
Classification: LCC R858 | NLM WA 950 | DDC 610.285–dc23 LC record available at http://lccn.loc.gov/2015039977

10 9 8 7 6 5 4 3 2 1

WORKBOOK TO ACCOMPANY INTRODUCTION TO BIOSTATISTICAL APPLICATIONS IN HEALTH RESEARCH WITH MICROSOFT® OFFICE EXCEL®

Contents

Preface

For many students of statistics, working out problems helps their understanding. For those students, I have written this workbook. For each chapter of the textbook there are several "Examples" with detailed answers. In addition, I have provided a summary of each chapter, a glossary, and a list of equations. These are intended to provide readers with a quick reference and as a means of review. Also for each chapter there are problems ("Exercises" with answers for only the odd exercises. The even exercises are problems that might be assigned for grading by your instructor.

The workbook has 13 chapters, but the text has only 12 chapters. The 13th chapter in the workbook addresses using the flowchart to select statistical methods for a given set of data. This chapter provides an overview of the textbook and its flowcharts.

Robert P. Hirsch

Acknowledgements

I gratefully acknowledge the role my students play in challenging me to help them to really understand statistical methods using more than just mathematical explanations.

Notices

The examples in this text are not intended to be a reflection of good clinical practice nor are they intended to provide information on use of medications. Some of the examples use data that have been created or modified to illustrate statistical methods.

CHAPTER 1

Thinking About Chance

CHAPTER SUMMARY

In Chapter 1 we learn that probabilities are useful in thinking about events (things that occur or characteristics that exist) relative to observations (opportunities for things to occur or characteristics to exist). When thinking about probabilities, we use literary, graphic, or mathematic language. In literary language, a probability is the frequency of events relative to the number of observations. In graphic language, we use Venn diagrams to think about probabilities. In Venn diagrams, a circular area usually represents occurrences of the event and a rectangle represents the observations. Then, the probability of the event is reflected by the area of the circle relative to the area of the rectangle. Mathematically, probabilities are proportions, because the number of events is part of the number of observations.

Workbook to Accompany Introduction to Biostatistical Applications in Health Research with Microsoft® Office Excel®, First Edition. Robert P. Hirsch.
© 2016 John Wiley & Sons, Inc. Published 2016 by John Wiley & Sons, Inc.

Regardless of which language we use to think about probabilities, we notice that probabilities have certain properties. One of these is that a probability must have a value within the range of zero to one. A probability of zero tells us that the event never occurs. A probability of one tells us that the event always occurs. Probabilities between zero and one tell us that the event sometimes occurs.

In addition to thinking about single events, we can use probabilities to think about collections of events. The first collection of events considered in Chapter 1 includes the event and its complement. The complement of an event includes everything that could happen in an observation except the event. Events and their complements always have two characteristics. One is that they are always collectively exhaustive. Events are collectively exhaustive when at least one of the events must occur in every observation. Another characteristic of events and their complements is that they are mutually exclusive. Being mutually exclusive means that, at most, only one of the events can occur in a particular observation.

We can have collections of events other than just a particular event and its complement. Other collections of events might be collectively exhaustive and/or mutually exclusive. An event and its complement, however, are always collectively exhaustive and mutually exclusive.

With other collections of events, we can be interested in two types relationships of the events. These are the intersection and the union of those events. In an intersection of events, we are interested in those observations in which all of the events occur. In a union of events, we are interested in those observations in which at least one of the events occurs.

When we are interested in the intersection of events, we can use the multiplication rule to calculate the probability of the intersection. There are two versions of the multiplication rule. The simplified version involves multiplying the probabilities of each event together. This simplified version is appropriate if the events are statistically independent (from each other). That is, if the probability of each event is the same regardless of whether the other event(s) occur(s). The full version of the multiplication rule uses conditional probabilities.

Many of the probabilities we encounter in health research and practice are conditional probabilities. What distinguishes conditional probabilities from other probabilities is the fact that conditional probabilities address a subset of the observations, rather than all of the observations. That subset of observations is specified by the conditioning event(s). The event(s) addressed by the conditional probability is specified by the conditional event(s). If events are statistically independent, then the probability of the conditional event occurring is the same regardless of whether the conditioning event occurs.

When we are interested in the union of events, we use the addition rule to calculate the probability of the union. There are two versions of the addition rule. In the simplified version, the probabilities of the events in the union are added together. This simplified version of the addition rule can be used when the events are mutually exclusive. If the events are not mutually exclusive, the probabilities of their intersections need to be taken into account.

The conditional and conditioning events in conditional probabilities have very different functions. A conditional probability addresses the probability that the conditional event(s) will occur under the assumption that the conditioning event(s) has occurred. Often we find we are interested in the probability that the conditioning event will occur assuming the conditional event has occurred. One example of this situation is the relationship among the probabilities used in interpreting diagnostic tests. Tests are characterized by their sensitivities and specificities. The conditioning events in sensitivity and specificity are whether or not a person has the disease. To interpret the result of a diagnostic test, however, we want to consider the probability that a person has the disease. In other words, we want to change whether someone has the disease from being the conditioning event to be the conditional event. The way in which we exchange conditional and conditioning events is by using Bayes' theorem.

GLOSSARY

Addition Rule – the method of calculating the union of two or more events. The simplified version involves adding the probabilities of the individual events together. The simplified version can be used if the events are mutually exclusive. The full version for the union of two events involves adding the probabilities of the events together and subtracting the probability of their intersection.

Bayes' Theorem – the mathematical description of the relationship between the probability of one event conditional on the occurrence of another event and the conditional probability of the second event conditional on the occurrence of the first event.

Chance – a process of producing events that has no apparent cause. For example, to say that chance affects whether or not a particular person in the population will be selected to be included in a sample, implies that we know of no characteristics of that person that make it more or less likely they will be selected. See Probability.

Collectively Exhaustive – a collection of events that includes all possible observations. For instance, being male or female is a collectively exhaustive set of genders.

Complement – (of an event) the occurrence of anything except the event. For example, if the event is being exposed to a particular carcinogen, the complement of that event is not being exposed to that carcinogen. An event and its complement are always mutually exclusive and collectively exhaustive.

Conditional Event – the particular event addressed by a conditional probability.

Conditional Probability – the chance that that a particular event will occur in an observation in which another event (or events) has occurred. For example, if we are interested in comparing the chance of getting a disease between persons who are either exposed or unexposed, a conditional probability of interest would be the probability of getting the disease given that a person is exposed.

Conditioning Event – the event that has occurred in an observation that influences the chance that the conditional event will occur in that same observation. For example, if we are interested in comparing the chance of getting a disease between persons who are either exposed or unexposed, the conditioning event would be exposure.

Event – something that happens or exists in an observation. Examples of events include being exposed, having a disease, being a woman, and being selected to be in a sample.

Frequency – how often something happens. For example, if there are 10 persons with a particular disease in a group of persons, the frequency of disease in the group is 10.

Independence – see Statistical Independence.

Intersection – observations that include all the events. For example, the intersection between being exposed and having a disease includes those persons who are both exposed and have the disease.

Multiplication Rule – the method of calculating the intersection of two or more events. The simplified version involves multiplying the probabilities of the individual events together. The simplified version can be used if the events are statistically independent. The full version for the intersection of two events involves multiplying the probability of one of the events by the probability of the other event, given that the first event occurs.

Mutually Exclusive – a collection of events in which only one event can occur in a given observation. For example, suppose that a disease has five stages and each person with the disease can only be in one of those stages. Then, the stages of that disease are mutually exclusive.

Observation – an opportunity for an event to occur. In health research, the most common observations are persons.

Probability – the chance that an event will occur. For example, the probability of someone developing a particular disease might be equal to 0.1. That implies that one-tenth of the observations will develop the disease. A probability is a proportion, so it can have values in the range of 0-1. See Chance and Proportion.

Proportion – a fraction in which the number in the numerator is also included in the denominator. A proportion has a discrete range of possible values ranging from zero to one.

Statistical Independence – a property of two (or more) events in which the probability of one event occurring is not affected by whether the other event (or events) has occurred. For example, if developing a disease and being exposed are statistically independent, the probability of developing the disease is the same regardless of whether a person is exposed.

Unconditional Probability – the probability of an event occurring regardless of whether another event has occurred. For example, the unconditional probability of developing a disease does not separate exposed from unexposed persons.

Union – observations which include one or more of a collection of events. For example, if we consider risk factors for breast cancer as a collection of events, the union of those risk factors includes persons who have at least one risk factor.

Venn Equations – a method of representing probabilities that combines graphic language (Venn diagram) and mathematic language (equation).

Venn Diagram – a graphic representation of the relationship between events and observations in which the area of a figure (usually a circle for events and a rectangle for observations) corresponds to the frequency of an event or observation. For example, a Venn diagram representing the occurrence of a disease would have a circle (representing persons with the disease) inside a rectangle (representing persons). The area of the circle relative to the area of the rectangle would be the same as the number of persons with the disease relative to the total number of persons.

EQUATIONS

$p(\overline{A}) = 1 - p(A)$

the probability of the complement of event A as it relates to the probability of event A. (see Equation{1.2})

$$p(A \text{ and } B) = p(A) \cdot p(B|A)$$
$$= p(B) \cdot p(A|B)$$

the probability of the intersection of events A and B. Either of the events can be represented by an unconditional probability. Then, the other event is represented by a conditional probability. This is the multiplication rule. (see Equation {1.4})

$p(A|B) = p(A|\overline{B}) = p(A)$

three probabilities that are equal to the same value if event A is statistically independent of event B. (see Equation {1.8})

$p(B|A) = \dfrac{p(A \text{ and } B)}{p(A)}$

the probability of event B given that event A occurs. (see Equation {1.9})

$p(A|B) = \dfrac{p(A \text{ and } B)}{p(B)}$

the probability of event A given that event B occurs.

$p(A \text{ and/or } B) =$
$p(A) + p(B) - p(A \text{ and } B)$

the probability of the union of events A and B. This is the addition rule. (see Equation {1.13})

$p(B|A) =$
$\dfrac{p(B) \cdot p(A|B)}{\left[p(B) \cdot p(A|B)\right] + \left[p(\overline{B}) \cdot p(A|\overline{B})\right]}$

the relationship between the probability of event B occurring given that event A occurs and the probability of event A occurring given that event B occurs. This is Bayes' theorem. (see Equation {1.18})

EXAMPLES

Suppose 25 persons who ate a buffet lunch at a particular restaurant developed salmonella infections (a type of food poisoning). As epidemiologists, we are interested in finding out what food from the buffet was associated with becoming ill. To investigate this, we ask the 25 persons who became ill (the cases), and another 100 persons who ate at the buffet, but did not become ill (the controls), what they ate. Imagine we observe the following results for the items offered that are most likely to be the source of the infection:

Table 1.1 Frequencies of eating different foods for cases and for controls.

FOOD	CASES	CONTROLS
Potato salad	10	40
Chicken salad	5	20
Egg salad	2	8
Seafood salad	5	20
Cole slaw	4	16
Deviled eggs	8	32
Turkey	12	18
Dressing	12	24
Chicken	10	40

Eating a particular food is considered an event.

1.1. Are these events mutually exclusive?

To be mutually exclusive, the probability of one event occurring given that another event has occurred must be equal to zero. In this context, mutual exclusion would mean that a person could not eat both turkey and dressing, for example. This is illustrated in Figure 1.1.

This is not likely to be true. Further, we can tell that at least some of the people ate more than one item. Among cases, the total number of items eaten is 68, but there are only 25 cases. Among the controls, the total number of items eaten is 218, but there are only 100 controls. The only explanation for those frequencies is that some people ate more than one item.

1.2. Are these events collectively exhaustive?

To be collectively exhaustive, all of the possible events must be listed. We are told that the listed items were "most likely to be the source of infection." This implies that there were other items on the buffet that were unlikely to cause a salmonella

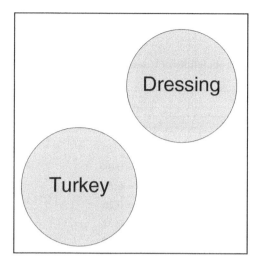

Figure 1.1.   Venn diagram illustrating mutual exclusion between eating turkey and eating dressing.

infection. If there were other items on the buffet, then the listed foods are not collectively exhaustive.

To determine which foods might be the source of the infection, we want look at the associations between each type of food eaten and becoming ill. An association between events is the same as the events not being statistically independent.

1.3. To look for statistical independence, what type of probabilities are going to be of primary interest? Why?

Statistical independence is defined by the relationship between conditional probabilities. If two events are statistically independent, then the probability of one event is the same regardless of whether another event occurs. Here, statistical independence means the probability of eating any particular item is the same for cases as it is for controls.

Next, we will change the data in Table 1 so that they reflect probabilities of eating each of the foods for cases and for controls.

1.4. What will be the numerator of those probabilities?

The numerator will be the number of cases eating a particular food or the number of controls eating a particular food.

1.5. What will be the denominator of those probabilities?

The denominator will be the number of cases or the number of controls.

1.6. Put the results of these calculations in a table.

Table 1.2 Probabilities of cases and controls eating particular foods.

FOOD	CASES	CONTROLS
Potato salad	$^{10}/_{25} = 0.40$	$^{40}/_{100} = 0.40$
Chicken salad	$^{5}/_{25} = 0.20$	$^{20}/_{100} = 0.20$
Egg salad	$^{2}/_{25} = 0.08$	$^{8}/_{100} = 0.08$
Seafood salad	$^{5}/_{25} = 0.20$	$^{20}/_{100} = 0.20$
Cole slaw	$^{4}/_{25} = 0.16$	$^{16}/_{100} = 0.16$
Deviled eggs	$^{8}/_{25} = 0.32$	$^{32}/_{100} = 0.32$
Turkey	$^{12}/_{25} = 0.48$	$^{18}/_{100} = 0.18$
Dressing	$^{12}/_{25} = 0.48$	$^{24}/_{100} = 0.24$
Chicken	$^{10}/_{25} = 0.40$	$^{40}/_{100} = 0.40$

1.7. What kind of probabilities are those in Table 1.2?

They are conditional probabilities with case or control as the conditioning event and eating a particular food as the conditional event.

1.8. If there is an association between eating a particular type of food and becoming ill, what relationship would we expect to see between the pairs of probabilities in Table 1.2?

If there is association between eating a particular type of food and becoming ill, then the conditional probabilities for that item will be unequal. Equal conditional probabilities are a sign of statistical independence, which is the same as no association.

1.9. For which food(s) is there an association with becoming ill?

The conditional probabilities for turkey and dressing are equal to different values for cases compared to controls. Cases had a higher probability of eating either of those foods than did controls.

1.10. Now, suppose no one ate both chicken and turkey. What do we call the relationship between those two events?

When the probability of one event is equal to zero if another event occurs, we call the events mutually exclusive.

Suppose we are interested in the probability that someone ate either turkey or chicken.

1.11. In what type of relationship between those events are we interested?

When we are interested in the probability of one and/or more events occurring, we are interested in the union of those events.

1.12. What is the probability that a case ate either turkey or chicken if no one ate both?

We find the union of two or more events by using the addition rule. When the events are mutually exclusive, we can use the simplified version of the addition rule.

$$p(\text{turkey or chicken}|\text{case}) = p(\text{turkey}|\text{case}) + p(\text{chicken}|\text{case}) = 0.48 + 0.40$$
$$= 0.88$$

Therefore, 88% of the cases ate either turkey or chicken.

1.13. What is the probability that a control ate either turkey or chicken if no one ate both?

Again, we are interested in the union of eating turkey and/or chicken. Since no one ate both, we can use the simplified version of the addition rule.

$$p(\text{turkey or chicken}|\text{control}) = p(\text{turkey}|\text{control}) + p(\text{chicken}|\text{control})$$
$$= 0.18 + 0.40 = 0.58$$

Therefore, 58% of the controls ate either turkey or chicken.

Now, suppose we are interested in how many people ate both potato salad and dressing.

1.14. In what type of relationship between those events are we interested?

When we are interested in both (all) events occurring in the same observation, we are interested in the intersection of the events.

1.15. If the probability of eating potato salad given that someone ate dressing is equal to 0.2 for both cases and controls, what is the probability that a case ate both potato salad and dressing?

Here, we are asked to calculate the probability of the intersection of eating potato salad and eating dressing for cases. We are told the probability of eating potato salad given that a case ate dressing is equal to 0.2. We know the events are not statistically independent since the conditional probability of eating potato salad is equal to 0.2, but the unconditional probability of eating potato salad among cases is 0.4 (from Table 2). Thus, we need to use the full version of the multiplication rule to calculate the probability of the intersection.

$$p(\text{Potato Salad and Dressing}) \;=\; p(\text{Dressing}) \cdot p(\text{Potato Salad}|\text{Dressing})$$
$$=\; 0.48 \cdot 0.2 = 0.096$$

1.16. What is the probability that a control ate both potato salad and dressing?

In this example, we are asked to calculate the probability of the intersection of eating potato salad and dressing among controls. The only difference between this example and the previous example is that we are considering controls. The conditional probability is the same for cases and controls, but the unconditional probability of eating dressing is different.

$$p(\text{Potato Salad and Dressing}) \;=\; p(\text{Dressing}) \cdot p(\text{Potato Salad}|\text{Dressing})$$
$$=\; 0.24 \cdot 0.2 = 0.048$$

EXERCISES

1.1. In a particular high school, 40 of the 200 graduating seniors report they have had unprotected sexual intercourse and 100 of the 200 graduating seniors report they have tried smoking marijuana at least once during high school. Further, 30 of the 100 graduating seniors who report they have tried smoking marijuana have also had unprotected sexual intercourse. Based on that information, which of the following is the best description of the relationship between having unprotected sexual intercourse and smoking marijuana?

A. Having unprotected sexual intercourse and smoking marijuana are not statistically independent but they are mutually exclusive.

B. Having unprotected sexual intercourse and smoking marijuana are statistically independent but they are not mutually exclusive.

C. Having unprotected sexual intercourse and smoking marijuana are both statistically independent and mutually exclusive.

D. Having unprotected sexual intercourse and smoking marijuana are neither statistically independent nor mutually exclusive.

E. There is not enough information given here to determine statistical independence and mutual exclusion of having unprotected sexual intercourse and smoking marijuana.

1.2. Suppose 25% of the children in a certain elementary school developed nausea and vomiting following a holiday party. None of the children who drank the apple cider at that party became ill. Based on that information, which of the following is the best description of the relationship between becoming ill and drinking apple cider at the party?

- **A.** Becoming ill and drinking cider are not statistically independent but they are mutually exclusive.
- **B.** Becoming ill and drinking cider are statistically independent but they are not mutually exclusive.
- **C.** Becoming ill and drinking cider are both statistically independent and mutually exclusive.
- **D.** Becoming ill and drinking cider are neither statistically independent nor mutually exclusive.
- **E.** There is not enough information given here to determine statistical independence and mutual exclusion of becoming ill and drinking cider.

1.3. In a particular population, 30% of the people smoke cigarettes and 10% of the people have chronic obstructive pulmonary disease (COPD). If having COPD is independent of smoking, what percent of the population would you expect to find who smoke and also have COPD?

- **A.** 0%
- **B.** 3%
- **C.** 10%
- **D.** 30%
- **E.** 40%

1.4. In a particular population, 5% of the infants have a low birthweight ($<2,500\,g$) and 60% of the mothers have at least 16 years of education. If having a mother with at least 16 years of education and having a low birthweight are statistically independent, which of the following is closest to the percentage of infants who have a mother with at least 16 years of education and who have a low birthweight?

- **A.** 0%
- **B.** 3%
- **C.** 6%
- **D.** 30%
- **E.** 40%

1.5. Suppose in a population of 10,000 persons, 5,000 smoke cigarettes and 7,500 have a high fat diet. Further, suppose that among the 5,000 persons who smoke cigarettes there are 3,000 who are also among the 7,500 who have a high fat diet. Based that information, which of the following is closest to the percentage of persons in the population who smoke cigarettes and/or have a high fat diet?

    A. 38%

    B. 50%

    C. 75%

    D. 88%

    E. 125%

1.6. In a particular population, 60% of infants receive only their mother's breast milk, 20% receive only commercial infant formula, and 20% receive both. What is the chance that a particular infant selected randomly would receive breast milk and/or formula?

    A. 0%

    B. 20%

    C. 80%

    D. 100%

    E. 120%

1.7. Suppose we are interested in the efficacy of a new treatment for anemia. To investigate this treatment, we randomly assign 50 persons with anemia to receive the new treatment and 50 persons with anemia to receive the standard treatment. Among those 100 persons, suppose 60% are cured. If there is no association between treatment and the chance of being cured, what percentage of the persons who received the new treatment would we expect to be cured?

    A. 0%

    B. 30%

    C. 36%

    D. 50%

    E. 60%

1.8. In a certain industry, 20% of the workers develop liver disease and 40% develop respiratory disease. If there is no association between developing liver disease and developing respiratory disease, what percentage of the workers who develop liver disease would we expect to develop respiratory disease?

    A. 0%

    B. 8%

    C. 20%

    D. 40%

    E. 100%

CHAPTER 2

Describing Populations

CHAPTER SUMMARY

In Chapter 2, we encounter distributions of data. A distribution of data is a description of how frequently various data values occur. In health research, we are interested in describing the distribution of data in the population. There are three ways we can do this. We can use literary language, graphic language, or mathematic language.

In literary language, we can describe a distribution of data by reporting which data values occur most frequently, less frequently, and least frequently. A literary description of a distribution of data is relatively easy to construct, but it leaves out quite a bit of detail about the distribution.

A better way to describe a distribution of data is using graphic language. There are several ways we can graphically describe a distribution; four of which are

Workbook to Accompany Introduction to Biostatistical Applications in Health Research with Microsoft® Office Excel®, First Edition. Robert P. Hirsch.
© 2016 John Wiley & Sons, Inc. Published 2016 by John Wiley & Sons, Inc.

introduced in Chapter 2. These are a bar graph, a histogram, a stem-and-leaf plot and a frequency polygon.

A bar graph is used to describe distributions of discrete data. Discrete data include ordinal and nominal data. Ordinal data are values that can be ordered in a meaningful way, but the spacing between the data values is not considered. Nominal data are values that describe groups that cannot be ordered in a meaningful way.

A bar graph has data values on the horizontal axis and either the frequency, proportion, or percent of each of the data values on the vertical axis. A bar is drawn for each data value, the height of which corresponds to the frequency, proportion, or percent of data values in the population equal to that specific value.

A histogram is used to describe continuous data. Continuous data have a large number of possible ordered values that are evenly-spaced.

A histogram is similar to a bar graph in that data values are on the horizontal axis; frequency, proportion, or percent is on vertical axis; and bars of various heights are used to represent the occurrence of the corresponding data values. There are two differences between a bar graph and a histogram. First, the bars in a histogram touch each other while there are spaces between the bars in a bar graph. This distinction reflects the differences between discrete data, in which there are spaces between data values and continuous data, in which (theoretically) there are no spaces between values.

The second distinction between a bar graph and a histogram is that the data values in a bar graph are specific values, while data values in a histogram are represented by intervals of values. This distinction is due to the fact that there are (theoretically) an infinite number of possible values for continuous data. If there are an infinite number of possible values, then the probability associated with any single value is essentially equal to zero. To have nonzero probabilities for continuous data, we need to think of intervals of values.

When we use histograms to describe a distribution of data, we need to decide how narrow the intervals will be. The narrower the intervals, the greater is the number of bars. As we approach an infinite number of bars that are infinitely narrow, the bars disappear. Then, we are left with just the tops of the bars that have the appearance of a line instead of a collection of bars. When we reach this point, we call the graph a frequency polygon.

The third graphic approach to describing distributions of data considered in this chapter is the stem-and-leaf plot. A stem-and-leaf plot is similar to a histogram, but it is easier to construct, especially when we graph relatively few data values. To begin, we put the left digit(s) for each value in a column. These are called the stem. Each of the components of the stem is like an interval of values in a histogram. Then, we list in a row following each component of the stem the right-most digit for each of the values that have that particular set of numbers to the left. These right-most digits are called the leaves. The result is like a histogram in which the number of leaves corresponds to the height of a bar in a histogram.

Most often, we use a mathematic description of the distribution of data in the population. To describe a distribution mathematically, we must first state the type of distribution and then, provide values for the parameters of the distribution. Parameters are numbers that designate a specific distribution of the stated type.

The type of distribution we considered, using the mathematic approach, was the Gaussian (or normal) distribution. The Gaussian distribution is a symmetric bell-shaped distribution. To specify a particular Gaussian distribution, we need to provide numeric values for two parameters. One parameter describes the location of the distribution in a continuum of values. The other parameter describes how dispersed the data are around that location.

The parameter of location for a Gaussian distribution is the mean. The mean can be thought of as the center of gravity of a distribution that reflects not only on which side of a distribution data values occur, but also how far away they are from the middle of the distribution. This is in contrast to the median, which reflects only on which side of the distribution data values occur.

The parameter of dispersion for a Gaussian distribution is the variance (or its square root: the standard deviation). The variance can be thought of as the mean of the squared differences between the data values and the mean of the distribution.

Once we can describe the distribution of data in the population, we can begin thinking about the role of chance in selecting a sample from that population. There are two ways we might do this. One of these is based on a graphic description of the distribution. The other is based on a mathematic description of the distribution.

The graphic approach is related to Venn diagrams and Venn equations examined in Chapter 1. Instead of a rectangle, all possible observations are represented by the entire distribution. For the events, we use the portion(s) of the distribution that corresponds to the values for which the probability is being calculated.

For the mathematic approach, we use the mathematic description of the distribution and the values of the parameters to calculate probabilities. Rather than do this for each distribution, these calculations have been performed for us and tabulated for standard distributions (see Appendix B). One of the standard distributions that can be used for a Gaussian distribution is called the standard normal distribution.

The standard normal distribution is a Gaussian distribution with a mean equal to zero and a standard deviation equal to one. When we want to calculate a probability for a datum from a Gaussian distribution, we can convert the mean of the distribution to a mean of zero by subtracting the actual mean from each data value. Then, we can convert the standard deviation to a value of one by dividing the difference between the mean and a data value by the actual standard deviation. We call the result a standard normal deviate or a z-value.

This process of converting a datum to a z-value determines what value on the standard normal scale corresponds to a particular value on the original scale. Then, we can determine the probability of an interval of values defined by that datum by determining the probability of an interval of values defined by the corresponding

z-value. To determine the probability for an interval of values defined by a z-value, we use a statistical table.

A statistical table for the standard normal distribution appears in Table B.1 of the textbook and this workbook. Table B.1 gives us the probabilities of getting a data value in an interval equal to the specific z-value or greater. This is called the upper tail of the distribution. In the standard normal distribution, the upper half of the distribution corresponds to positive z-values. The lower half of the distribution does not appear in Table B.1, but the standard normal distribution is a symmetric distribution centered on zero, so what is true for a positive value or more is the same as what is true for a negative value or less. To find probabilities for intervals of values in the middle of the standard normal distribution, we determine the probabilities for the tails excluded by the interval and subtract the probability from one.

GLOSSARY

Bar Graph – a graph used to describe a distribution of discrete data. Data values appear on the horizontal axis and frequency, proportion, or percent appear on the vertical axis. The height of a bar corresponding to specific data value reflects how often that data value occurs. The bars in a bar graph do not touch as an indication that there are gaps between possible data values.

Continuous Data – data with a large number of possible values that are ordered and evenly-spaced. Examples of continuous data include weight, height, blood pressure, age, and serum cholesterol. Antonym: Discrete Data.

Data – information. Anything that can be measured or observed. Singular: Datum

Discrete Data – data with a limited number of values between which there are no possible values. Examples of discrete data include ordinal data such as level of agreement and stage of disease and nominal data such as country of origin and gender. Antonym: Continuous Data.

Dispersion – how spread out data values are around some location.

Distribution – a description of how frequently various data values occur.

Frequency Polygon – a graphic representation of the distribution of continuous data. A frequency polygon results from increasing the number of bars in a histogram to infinity.

Gaussian Distribution – a symmetric, bell-shaped curve with data near the middle of the distribution occurring most frequently and data toward the extremes occurring more and more rarely as the distance from the middle increases. Synonym: Normal Distribution

Histogram – a graphic representation of the distribution of continuous data in which bars are used to represent the frequency (or proportion or percent) of values (represented on the vertical axis) within specified intervals of data (represented on the horizontal axis). The bars in a histogram touch each other as an indication that there are no gaps in possible values between the intervals.

Interquartile Range (IQR) – a measure of dispersion that is not affected by spacing between data values. The IQR is found by dividing the data values in half by determining the median and, then, dividing each half in half using the medians of the halves. The IQR is the distance between the median of the lower half and the median of the upper half. The IQR can be used to calculate the standard deviation of continuous data that occur in a Gaussian distribution.

Location – a point in a distribution around which the data values are centered.

Mean – the center of gravity of a distribution that is influenced by to which side and how far away data values are from the middle of the distribution. The mean is the parameter of location of a Gaussian distribution.

Median – the physical center of a distribution with half the data values occurring above it and half the data values occurring below it. Unlike the mean, the distance from the center of the distribution at which data values occur does not affect their influence on the value of the median.

Mode – the most frequently occurring data value in a distribution. A distribution can have no mode, one mode, or more than one mode.

Nominal Data – data values that cannot be ordered in a meaningful way. Nominal data also include any data with only two possible values (even if they can be ordered). Examples of nominal data include country of origin, gender, names of medications, discharge diagnoses, and blood type.

One-Tailed (One-Sided) Probability – the probability associated with one of the extremes of a distribution (i.e., high values or low values, but not both).

Ordinal Data – data values that can be ordered, in which the spacing between values is not considered. Examples of ordinal data include level of agreement, stage of disease, and Apgar score.

Parameter – a number that describes the distribution in the population. Gaussian distributions have two parameters: the mean (specifying location) and variance or standard deviation (specifying dispersion).

Population – collection of all possible data values. This is the group that research is intended to address.

Range – difference between the highest and lowest data values. The range is sometimes used to reflect the dispersion of a distribution.

Skewed Distribution – a distribution with more data values at one extreme than at the other extreme. Synonym: Asymmetric Distribution

Standard Deviation – the square root of the variance.

Standard Normal Deviate – a value from the standard normal distribution. Synonym: z-value.

Standard Normal Distribution – a Gaussian distribution with a mean of zero and a standard deviation of one.

Statistical Table – usually refers to a table that provides probabilities associated with various values of a standard distribution.

Stem-and-Leaf Plot – a graphic method of describing a distribution of continuous data. The "stem" is made up of all but the rightmost digit of each number and the "leaves" are the rightmost digits. A stem-and-leaf plot is easy to construct without using a graphics program. It looks like the mirror image of a histogram rotated 90 degrees.

Two-Tailed (or Two-sided) Probability – the probability associated with both of the extremes of a distribution (i.e., high values and low values).

Variance – the parameter of dispersion of a Gaussian distribution. The variance is the mean of the squared differences between each data value and the mean.

EQUATIONS

$\mu = \dfrac{\sum Y_i}{N}$ mean of the distribution of data in the population. (see Equation {2.1})

$\sigma^2 = \dfrac{\sum (Y_i - \mu)^2}{N}$ variance of the distribution of data in the population. (see Equation{2.3})

$\sigma = \sqrt{\sigma^2}$ standard deviation of the distribution of data in the population calculated from the variance. (see Equation{2.4})

$\sigma = \frac{2}{3} IQR$ standard deviation of the distribution of data in the population calculated from the interquartile range. (see Equation{2.5})

$z = \dfrac{Y_i - \mu}{\sigma}$ conversion of a datum to a standard normal deviate (i.e., z-value). (see Equation{2.6})

EXAMPLES

Suppose we are studying births in a certain population and we measure birth weight, birth order, gender, mother's race, and mother's age.

2.1. Indicate the type of data for each measurement taken in the study.

Table 2.1   Types of data

MEASUREMENT	TYPE OF DATA
Birth weight	Continuous (large number of evenly-spaced values)
Birth order	Ordinal (spacing unknown)
Gender	Nominal (two groups of unordered values)
Mother's race	Nominal (limited number of groups with unordered values)
Mother's age	Continuous (large number of evenly-spaced values)

In Table 2.2 the percent of births according mothers' race are listed.

Table 2.2   Percent births in a certain population according to mother's race

RACE	Percent
African American	30%
Asian	10%
Hispanic	35%
Native American	5%
White	20%

2.2. Describe the distribution of births according to race graphically.

Since these are discrete data, we select "column chart" in Excel[1]

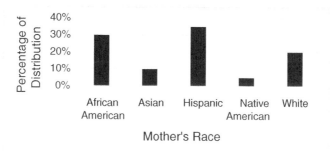

Figure 2.1.   Bar graph of mother's race

Table 2.3 lists birthweights in a certain population.

Table 2.3   Percent of births according to birth weight (gm)

BIRTH WEIGHT	PERCENT
1,500–1,749	1%
1,750–1,999	2%
2,000–2,249	5%
2,250–2,499	11%
2,500–2,749	15%
2,750–2,999	26%
3,000–3,249	17%
3,250–3,499	10%
3,500–3,749	8%
3,750–3,999	3%
4,000–4,249	1%
4,250–4,499	1%

[1] You can create graphics in Excel by selecting the Insert tab, then selecting the kind of chart you desire.

2.3. Describe the distribution of birth weights graphically.

Birth weights are continuous data, so we want to use a histogram to describe them. We can get a histogram by selecting "column chart," right-clicking on one of the bars, and selecting "Format Data Series." Then, click on the column chart icon and set the "Gap Width" to zero.

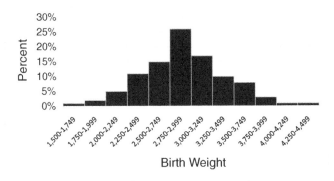

Figure 2.2. Histogram of birth weights

2.4. What is the probability that an infant in the population will have a birth weight of less than 2,000 gm?

To determine a probability, we sum the percentages (or proportions) that satisfy the criterion. For birth weight less than 2,000 gm, we add the 1,500–1,749 and 1,750–1,999 category percentages.

$$p(< 2,000) = 1\% + 2\% = 3\%$$

2.5. What is the probability that an infant in the population will have a birth weight of at least 2,000 gm but less than 3,500 gm?

To determine the probability for a wide range of values, it is sometimes easier to find the complement of the probabilities of the excluded part of the distribution.

$$p(\geq 2,000 \text{ and } < 3,500) = 100\% - p(< 2,000 \text{ or } \geq 3,500)$$
$$= 100\% - (1\% + 2\% + 8\% + 3\% + 1\% + 1\%) = 84\%$$

Now, let us assume the distribution of birth weights is a Gaussian distribution with a mean equal to 2,900 gm and a variance equal to 250,000 gm.

2.6. What standard normal deviate corresponds to a birth weight of 3,600 gm?

We find the standard normal deviate (z-value), by subtracting the mean and dividing by the standard deviation.

$$z = \frac{Y_i - \mu}{\sigma} = \frac{3,600 - 2,900}{\sqrt{250,000}} = 1.40$$

2.7. What is the probability of getting a standard normal deviate equal to or less than 1.40?

To find probabilities related to specific standard normal deviates, we use Table B1. The probabilities in Table B1 are in the upper tail of the standard normal distribution (or in the lower tail for the negative equivalent of the z-value).

$$p(z \geq 1.40) = 0.0808$$
$$p(z \leq 1.40) = 1 - 0.0808 = 0.9192$$

2.8. What is the probability an infant in the population will have a birth weight of at least 3.600 gm?

A z-value of 1.40 in the standard normal distribution corresponds to a birth weight of 3,600 gm, so the probability of a birth weight equal to or greater than 3,600 gm is the same as the probability of a z-value of 1.40 or larger found in previous example.

$$p(BW \geq 3,600) = p(z \geq 1.40) = 0.0808$$

2.9. What is the probability an infant in the population will have a birth weight of exactly 3,600 gm?

The answer is zero! This is a trick question designed to emphasize that the probability of any specific value in a continuum is essentially equal to zero. The reason for this is there are, at least theoretically, an infinite number of possible values. Any number divided by infinity is essentially equal to zero.

2.10. What is the probability an infant in the population will have a birth weight of at least 2,100?

The answer to this question involves two steps. First, we need to find what z-value corresponds to a birth weight of 2,100 gm. Then, we need to find what probability is associated with the z-value. For the first step, we get:

$$z = \frac{Y_i - \mu}{\sigma} = \frac{2,100 - 2,900}{\sqrt{250,000}} = -1.60$$

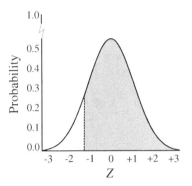

Figure 2.3. $z = -1.60$ or more

The probability associated with 1.60 or more is 0.0548, so the probability of 2,100 or more is 1.0000–0.0548 = 0.9452.

EXERCISES

2.1. In a particular population, the mean birth weight is equal to 3,500 grams and the standard deviation of birth weights is equal to 800 grams. Given that information, and assuming that birth weight has a Gaussian distribution, which of the following is closest to the probability that an infant selected randomly will weigh between 3000 and 4000 grams?

   A. 0.2676

   B. 0.4648

   C. 0.5352

   D. 0.7324

   E. 0.9175

2.2. Suppose we are interested in the length of gestation among live births in a particular population. If the mean gestation period is equal to 38 weeks and the standard deviation is equal to 1 week, and if we assume the distribution of gestational age is a Gaussian distribution, which of the following is closest to the probability that any given pregnancy will last longer than 38 weeks?

   A. 0.0228

   B. 0.0456

   C. 0.5000

   D. 0.9544

   E. 0.9772

2.3. In a particular population, the mean age is 45 years and the variance of age is equal to 225 years^2. Given that information, and assuming age has a Gaussian distribution, what is the probability a person selected randomly will be between 30 and 60 years of age?

A. 0

B. 0.1587

C. 0.3174

D. 0.6826

E. 0.8413

2.4. The mean systolic blood pressure in a particular population is 130 mmHg and has a standard deviation of 20 mmHg. Hypertension is considered severe if a patient has a systolic blood pressure equal to or greater than 180 mmHg. Given that information, and assuming that the distribution of systolic blood pressures is a Gaussian distribution, what percent of the population would have severe hypertension?

A. 0.6%

B. 2.0%

C. 6.0%

D. 17.1%

E. 20.2%

2.5. Consider a population in which the mean systolic blood pressure is 130 mmHg with a standard deviation of 20 mmHg. People with systolic blood pressure between 140 mmHg and 180 mmHg are considered to have mild to moderate hypertension. Given that information, and assuming that the distribution of systolic blood pressures is a Gaussian distribution, what percent of the population would have mild to moderate hypertension?

A. 3.0%

B. 3.3%

C. 30.2%

D. 43.8%

E. 67.1%

2.6. Consider a population in which the mean systolic blood pressure is 130 mmHg with a standard deviation of 20 mmHg. People with systolic blood pressure below 90 mmHg are considered to have hypotension. Given that information, and assuming that the distribution of systolic blood pressures is a Gaussian distribution, what percent of the population would have hypotension?

A. 2.3%

B. 4.6%

C. 24.3%

D. 45.4%

E. 47.7%

CHAPTER 3

Examining Samples

CHAPTER SUMMARY

In Chapter 3, we learned how to draw inferences about the population by examining a sample's observations. There are two processes that we can use. The first of these is estimation. In the process of estimation, the goal is to guess about the value of a parameter in the population. There are two kinds of estimates we use. One of those is a point estimate. A point estimate is a single number that is our best guess at the value of the parameter. The problem with point estimates is that they have a very low chance of being exactly equal to the population's parameter. This is because there are so many possible values that the probability for any single value is close to zero.

The other kind of estimate is an interval estimate, which is also known as a confidence interval. It differs from a point estimate in that an interval estimate

Workbook to Accompany Introduction to Biostatistical Applications in Health Research with Microsoft® Office Excel®, First Edition. Robert P. Hirsch.
© 2016 John Wiley & Sons, Inc. Published 2016 by John Wiley & Sons, Inc.

implies that the population's parameter lies within an interval of values. The width of an interval estimate determines the level of confidence we can have that the population's parameter is included in the interval. The most commonly used interval estimate gives us 95% confidence that the parameter is included. In addition to the selected level of confidence, the width of an interval estimate is affected by the precision with which we can estimate the parameter. The greater the precision, the narrower the interval.

The second process we can use to draw inferences about the population by examining a sample is statistical hypothesis testing. In statistical hypothesis testing, we begin with a hypothesis that makes a specific statement about the population. This hypothesis is called the null hypothesis. It is so named because a specific statement that has a relevant biologic interpretation usually says that nothing is different. The next step is to take a sample from the population. It is important to note, in statistical hypothesis testing, the hypothesis comes before the data are collected.

Most of the "work" in statistical hypothesis testing involves calculations necessary to determine the P-value. A P-value is a conditional probability. The conditional event is getting a sample at least as different from what the null hypothesis states as the sample we observed. The conditioning event is that the null hypothesis is true. It is important not to get these events interchanged. A P-value does not tell us the probability that the null hypothesis is true. Instead, the P-value assumes that it is true.

The final step in hypothesis testing is deciding what to conclude. Our conclusion depends on how the numeric magnitude of the P-value compares to some preselected value called alpha (α). The most usual value of alpha is 0.05. If the P-value is less than or equal to alpha, we reject the null hypothesis. That is to say, we conclude that the null hypothesis is not a true statement about the population.

When we reject the null hypothesis, we automatically accept the alternative hypothesis as true. The alternative hypothesis is not tested. It is considered to be true whenever the null hypothesis is considered to be false. For this to work, the null and alternative hypotheses must cover all possibilities for the population. Keeping this in mind is important when choosing between a two-sided (in which differences from the null hypothesis can occur in both directions) and a one-sided (in which differences from the null hypothesis can occur in only one direction) alternative hypothesis. Most often, two-sided alternative hypotheses are the appropriate choice.

There are two kinds of errors that can be made in hypothesis testing. A type I error occurs when the null hypothesis is rejected but it is, in fact, true. The chance of making a type I error is determined by the choice of the value of alpha. If alpha is equal to 0.05, there is a 0.05 chance of making a type I error. A type II error occurs when the null hypothesis is accepted as true but it is, in fact, false. We do not know the probability of making a type II error, since the alternative hypothesis does not make a specific statement about the population. Because we do not know the chance of making a type II error, we avoid any opportunity for this type of error to occur. We do this by refusing to conclude that the null hypothesis is true. When the P-value is larger than alpha, we do not accept the null hypothesis as being true. Instead, we refrain from drawing a conclusion about the null hypothesis. This is often referred to as "failing to reject" the null hypothesis.

Both interval estimation and hypothesis testing take into account the role of chance in selecting a sample from the population. In Chapter 2, we considered this role of chance in selecting an individual from the population by using the distribution of data. When we are taking the role of chance on the entire sample, we use a different distribution. This distribution is called the sampling distribution. It is the distribution of estimates from all possible samples of a given size.

An important feature of the sampling distribution is that is tends to be a Gaussian distribution, even if the distribution of data is not a Gaussian distribution. This is especially true of sampling distributions of estimates of parameters of location from larger samples. This principle is called the central limit theorem. It is because of the central limit theorem that many of the statistical procedures commonly used in analyzing health research data are based on Gaussian distributions.

The parameters of the sampling distribution are related to the parameters of the distribution of data. The means of the two distributions are equal to the same value. This will always be the case for any unbiased estimate. An unbiased estimate is equal to the population's parameter, on the average. This is reflected in the sampling distribution by having the mean equal to the parameter that is being estimated (i.e., mean of the distribution of data).

The variances and standard deviations of the sampling distribution and distribution of data are related, but not equal to the same value. The sampling distribution is less dispersed than is the distribution of data. The reason for this is that the impact of extreme data values in a sample is offset by less extreme data values. Thus, estimates of the mean have less variation than do the data. How much less, depends on the number of observations in the sample. The greater the number of observations, the less variable the estimates. To emphasize the difference in dispersion between the sampling distribution and the distribution of data, the standard deviation of the sampling distribution is usually called the standard error.

Both interval estimation and hypothesis testing use the sampling distribution to take into account the role of chance in selecting a sample from the population. In hypothesis testing, it is the sampling distribution that is used to calculate a P-value. In interval estimation, it is the standard error of the sampling distribution that is used to represent the precision with which the parameter has been estimated. Although these sound like different processes, they are really just mirror images of the same logical procedure. If a null hypothesis is rejected, the null value will be outside the limits of the confidence interval.[1] If the null value is inside the confidence interval, the null hypothesis would not be rejected. This relationship allows us to use confidence intervals to test null hypotheses.

---

[1] Being exactly equal to the limit of a confidence interval is considered to be outside the interval.

GLOSSARY

Alpha (α) – in statistical hypothesis testing, alpha is the probability of making a type I error, because it is the value that the *P*-value must be equal to or less than to reject the null hypothesis. In interval estimation, alpha is the complement of the level of confidence we have that the population's parameter is included in the confidence interval.

Alternative Hypothesis – a statement concerning the population that must be true if the null hypothesis is not true. The alternative hypothesis and the null hypothesis are a collectively exhaustive set of possibilities for the population. In other words, one of those two hypotheses must be true.

Beta (β) – in statistical hypothesis testing, beta is the probability of making a type II error.

Central Limit Theorem – the statement that sampling distributions for estimates of parameters of location (such as the mean) tend to be Gaussian distributions, even if the data do not come from a Gaussian distribution. This tendency is greater for larger samples.

Confidence Interval – see Interval Estimate.

Degrees of Freedom – when used in calculation of an estimate of variance, degrees of freedom are the amount of information a sample contains to make the estimate.

Estimate – a value calculated from the sample's observations as a guess at the value of the population's parameter. See Point Estimate, Interval Estimate.

Estimation – the process of calculating a guess at the value of a parameter in the population from the observations in a sample.

Hypothesis testing – a process of drawing inferences about the population based on an examination of the sample's observations. Statistical hypothesis testing is a deductive process that begins with the formation of the null hypothesis and draws a conclusion based on the likelihood that the sample came from a population in which the null hypothesis was true.

Interval Estimate – an interval of values within which there is a good chance (most often, a 95% chance) that the population's value occurs. Synonym: Confidence Interval.

Null Hypothesis – a specific statement about the population that is tested in statistical hypothesis testing.

Null Value – the value of the population's parameter according to the null hypothesis.

One-Sided – when chance is taken into account by considering only one tail of the sampling distribution. A one-sided confidence interval has a finite limit in only one direction (i.e., above or below the point estimate). A one-sided alternative hypothesis considers possibilities in only one direction (i.e., either above or below the null value). Synonym: One-tailed.

P-value – the probability of getting a sample at least as far from the null value as is the sample's estimate given that the null hypothesis is true. The *P*-value is calculated as part of statistical hypothesis testing. It is compared to alpha to decide whether or not to reject the null hypothesis.

Point Estimate – a single value calculated from the sample's observations that is the best guess at the value of a parameter in the population.

Sample – a subset of the data from a population that we examine in an attempt to describe the population.

Sampling Distribution – the theoretical distribution of estimates that would be observed if all possible samples of a given size were selected from the population. It is the sampling distribution that is used to take into account the influence of chance on an estimate.

Standard Error – the standard deviation of a sampling distribution.

Statistically Significant – the result of statistical hypothesis testing is said to be statistically significant if the null hypothesis can be rejected.

Two-sided – when chance is taken into account by considering both tails of the sampling distribution. A two-sided confidence interval has finite limits in both directions (i.e., above and below the point estimate). A two-sided alternative hypothesis considers possibilities in both directions (i.e., above and below the null value). Synonym: Two-tailed.

Type I Error – mistakenly rejecting a true null hypothesis.

Type II Error – mistakenly accepting a false null hypothesis.

Unbiased – the property of a method of estimation in which the estimates from repeated samples are equal to the population's parameter, on the average.

EQUATIONS

$$\mu \triangleq \overline{Y} = \frac{\sum Y_i}{n}$$

sample's point estimate of the mean of the distribution of data in the population. (see Equation {3.2})

$$\sigma^2 \triangleq s^2 = \frac{\sum (Y_i - \overline{Y})^2}{n-1}$$

sample's point estimate of the variance of the distribution of data in the population. (see Equation {3.4})

$$s = \sqrt{s^2}$$

sample's point estimate of the standard deviation of the distribution of data in the population. (see Example 3-1)

$$\mu_{\overline{Y}} = \mu \triangleq \overline{Y}$$

sample's point estimate of the mean of the sampling distribution for estimates of the mean. (see Equation {3.5})

$$\sigma_{\overline{Y}}^2 = \frac{\sigma^2}{n} \triangleq \frac{s^2}{n}$$

sample's point estimate of the variance of the sampling distribution for estimates of the mean (the square of the standard error). (see Equation {3.6})

$$\sigma_{\bar{Y}} = \sqrt{\frac{\sigma^2}{n}} \triangleq s_{\bar{Y}} = \sqrt{\frac{s^2}{n}} \text{ or } \frac{s}{\sqrt{n}}$$ sample's point estimate of the standard error (i.e., the standard deviation of the sampling distribution) for estimates of the mean. (see Equation {3.7})

$$\mu \triangleq \bar{Y} \pm (z_{\alpha/2} \cdot \sigma_{\bar{Y}})$$ sample's interval estimate (i.e., confidence interval) of the mean of the distribution of data in the population. (see Equation {3.8})

$$z = \frac{\bar{Y} - \mu_0}{\sigma_{\bar{Y}}}$$ conversion of the sample's estimate of the mean to a standard normal deviate (i.e., z-value). (see Equation {3.10})

EXAMPLES

In Chapter 2, we were interested in birth weights of infants in a particular population in which the mean birth weight is equal to 2,900 grams and the variance of birth weights is equal to 250,000 grams^2. Now, suppose we take a sample of 10 births from that population and observe the following results:

Table 3.1   Birth weights for a sample of 10 births.

Y	$Y - \bar{Y}$	$(Y - \bar{Y})^2$
2,950	−7	49
3,010	53	2,809
2,895	−62	3,844
3,110	153	23,409
3,055	98	9,604
3,185	228	51,984
3,000	43	1,849
2,660	−297	88,209
2,945	−12	144
2,760	−197	38,809
TOTAL 29,570	0	220,710

3.1. Calculate the sample's estimates of the mean and variance of birth weights in the population.

Most of the work in calculating these by hand has been done for us. We have the sum of the data values for calculation of the mean and the sum of squares for calculation of the variance.

$$\mu \triangleq \bar{Y} = \frac{\sum Y_i}{n} = \frac{29,570}{10} = 2,957 \text{ gm}$$

$$\sigma^2 \triangleq s^2 = \frac{\sum (Y_i - \bar{Y})^2}{n - 1} = \frac{220,710}{10 - 1} = 24,523.3 \text{ gm}^2$$

3.2. Calculate the sample's estimate of the standard error.

The sample's estimate of the standard error of the mean is calculated from the sample's estimate of the variance as follows:

$$\sigma_{\bar{Y}} \stackrel{\Delta}{=} s_{\bar{Y}} = \sqrt{\frac{s^2}{n}} = \sqrt{\frac{24,523.3}{10}} = 49.5 \text{ gm}$$

3.3. Use Excel to estimate the mean, variance, and standard error. How do these compare to the answers to the first two examples?

To obtain estimates of the mean, variance, and standard error, we use the "Descriptive Statistics" analysis tool in "Data Analysis" under the "Data" tab.

Column1	
Mean	2957
Standard Error	49.5210393
Median	2975
Mode	#N/A
Standard Deviation	156.5992763
Sample Variance	24523.33333
Kurtosis	0.253613234
Skewness	--0.632190736
Range	525
Minimum	2660
Maximum	3185
Sum	29570
Count	10
Confidence Level(95.0%)	112.0243738

The mean, variance, and standard error are the same as the rounded values we got when calculating these values by hand.
   Now, suppose the population's standard error is equal to the sample's estimate $(\sigma_{\bar{Y}} = s_{\bar{Y}})$.

3.4. Calculate a 95%, two-sided, confidence interval for the mean birth weight in this population.

To calculate a 95%, two-sided confidence interval for the mean, we need the point estimate of the mean and the standard error. We also need a z-value from Table B.1 to represent 95% confidence split between the tails of the standard normal distribution. That z-value is equal to 1.96.

$$\mu \stackrel{\Delta}{=} \bar{Y} \pm (z_{\alpha/2} \cdot \sigma_{\bar{Y}}) = 2,957 \pm (1.96 \cdot 49.5) = 2,859.9 \text{ to } 3,054.1$$

3.5. Use Excel to calculate a 95%, two-sided, confidence interval for the mean birth weight in the population. How does this interval compare to the answer to the previous example?

We can get the information we need for the confidence interval from the "Descriptive Statistics" analysis tool in "Data Analysis." In that output, we are given a number labeled as "Confidence Level (95.0%)." To obtain a 95% confidence interval, we add and subtract this value from the point estimate of the mean. The limits of that confidence interval are 2,845.0 and 3,069. This is a wider confidence interval than the one we calculated in the previous example. The difference between these confidence intervals will be the subject of Chapter 4.

Suppose we wonder if this population is actually a sample from a larger population in which the mean birth weight is equal to 3,000 grams. To address this possibility, we could test the null hypothesis that the mean birth weight in the population from which this sample was taken is equal to 3,000 grams.

3.6. What would be the appropriate alternative hypothesis?

The null hypothesis is the mean in the population is equal to 3,000 gm. The alternative hypothesis must hypothesize that the mean in the population is equal to any other possible value, except the value in the null hypothesis. There is no reason to believe there are impossible values, so the alternative hypothesis is that the mean is not equal to 3,000 gm.

3.7. Test that null hypothesis while allowing a 5% chance of rejecting the null hypothesis if that null hypothesis was true.

To test the null hypothesis that the mean birth weight in the population is equal to 3,000 gm, we convert the observed mean to a standard normal deviate.[2]

$$z = \frac{2,957 - 3,000}{49.5} = -0.87$$

To obtain the P-value, we look up −0.87 in Table B.1. In that table, we learn a standard normal deviate of −0.87 corresponds to a probability of 0.1922 in each tail of the standard normal distribution. Thus, the P-value is two times 0.1922 or 0.3844. Since this P-value is greater than 0.05, we fail to reject the null hypothesis (i.e., we remain inconclusive).

3.8. How could you have tested that null hypothesis using the confidence interval from a previous example?

An easier way to test the null hypothesis that the mean birth weight is equal to 3,000 gm in the population, if we have a confidence interval, is to determine

---

[2] We will learn a better method in Chapter 4.

whether the null value (3,000 gm) is included within or excluded from the confidence interval (2,859.9 to 3,054.1). Since the null value is included in this interval, we fail to reject the null hypothesis.

EXERCISES

3.1. Suppose we were to take a sample of 10 births from a given population and determine the gestational ages (in days) at birth. Imagine that we observe the following results: 266, 267, 256, 259, 261, 255, 270, 271, 269, 266. Create an Excel dataset using those observations. What is the point estimate of the mean gestational age in the population from which this sample was drawn?

    A. 220

    B. 225

    C. 255

    D. 264

    E. 306

3.2. Suppose we were to take a sample of 10 births from a given population and determine the gestational ages (in days) at birth. Imagine that we observe the following results: 266, 267, 256, 259, 261, 255, 270, 271, 269, 266. Create an Excel dataset using those observations. What is the sample's estimate of the standard deviation of gestational age in the population from which this sample was drawn?

    A. 2.6

    B. 3.1

    C. 3.4

    D. 4.3

    E. 5.8

3.3. Suppose we are interested in diastolic blood pressure (dbp) among persons in a particular population. To investigate this, we take a sample of 9 persons from the population and measure their dbp. Imagine we obtain the following results 75, 80, 81, 72, 85, 88, 91, 87, 88. Create an Excel dataset using those observations. Which of the following is closest to the sample's estimate of the variance of diastolic blood pressure values?

    A. 6.4

    B. 17.5

    C. 41.5

    D. 74.7

    E. 83.0

3.4. Suppose we take a sample of 36 persons from a particular population and measure their body weight. Then, we give each person a one-month's supply of appetite suppressants. At the end of the month, we weigh each person again and subtract their new weight from their first weight. Suppose we observe a mean difference in weight equal to 10 kg and we know the variance of differences in weight in the population is equal to 900 kg^2. Which of the following is closest to the interval of values within which we have 95% confidence that the population's mean lies?

    A. 0.0 to 20.0

    B. 0.2 to 19.8

    C. 2.3 to 17.7

    D. 5.0 to 15.0

    E. 8.0 to 12.0

3.5. Suppose we were to conduct a study in which 16 persons with hypothyroidism were given two medications in a random order. In this study, we measure TSH (thyroid stimulating hormone) after the participants had taken each of the medications for a week. Suppose we observe that the mean difference in TSH levels was equal to 20 mg/dL and we know the standard deviation of differences between TSH levels is equal to 60 mg/dL in the population. Which of the following is closest to the value that reflects the precision with which we will be able to estimate the mean from that sample's observations (i.e., the standard error)?

    A. 1.9

    B. 3.7

    C. 5.0

    D. 7.7

    E. 15.0

3.6. Suppose we were to conduct a study in which 16 persons with hypothyroidism were given two medications in a random order. In this study, we measure TSH after the participants had taken each of the medications for a week. Suppose we estimate the mean difference in TSH levels to be equal to 20 mg/dL and we estimate the standard deviation of differences between TSH levels to be equal to 60 mg/dL. What is the best null hypothesis to test about the mean difference in the population?

    A. $\mu = 0$

    B. $\mu > 0$

    C. $\mu < 0$

    D. $\mu \neq 0$

    E. $\mu = ?$

3.7. Suppose we were to conduct a study in which 16 persons with hypo-thyroidism were given two medications in a random order. In this study, we measure TSH after the participants had taken each of the medications for a week. Suppose we estimate the mean difference in TSH levels to be equal to 20 mg/dL and we estimate the standard deviation of differences between TSH levels to be equal to 60 mg/dL. What is the best alternative hypothesis to consider about the mean difference in the population?

A. $\mu = 0$

B. $\mu > 0$

C. $\mu < 0$

D. $\mu \neq 0$

E. $\mu = ?$

3.8. Suppose we were to conduct a study in which 16 persons with hypo-thyroidism were given two medications in a random order. In this study, we measure TSH after the participants had taken each of the medications for a week. Suppose we estimate the mean difference in TSH levels to be equal to 20 mg/dL and we estimate the standard deviation of differences between TSH levels to be equal to 60 mg/dL. Test the appropriate null hypothesis allowing a 5% chance of making a type I error. Which of the following is the best conclusion to draw?

A. Reject the null hypothesis

B. Accept the null hypothesis

C. Fail to reject the null hypothesis

D. Fail to accept the null hypothesis

E. Hypothesis testing is not appropriate for these data

3.9. Suppose we take a sample of 36 persons from a particular population and measure their body weight. Then, we give each person a one-month's supply of appetite suppressants. At the end of the month, we weigh each person again and subtract their new weight from their first weight. Suppose we observe a mean difference in weight equal to 10 kg and calculate a 95% confidence interval for the estimate that ranges from 0.2 kg to 19.8 kg. Which of the following are the best null and alternative hypotheses to test about the mean difference in the population?

A. H_0: $\mu = 0$ and H_A: $\mu = 0$

B. H_0: $\mu \neq 0$ and H_A: $\mu = 0$

C. H_0: $\mu = 0$ and H_A: $\mu \neq 0$

D. H_0: $\mu = 0$ and H_A: $\mu > 0$

E. H_0: $\mu = 0$ and H_A: $\mu < 0$

3.10. Suppose we take a sample of 36 persons from a particular population and measure their body weight. Then, we give each person a one-month's supply of appetite suppressants. At the end of the month, we weigh each person again and subtract their new weight from their first weight. Suppose we observe a mean difference in weight equal to 10 kg and calculate a 95% confidence interval for that estimate that ranges from 0.2 kg to 19.8 kg. Which of the following is the best conclusion to draw if we were to test the null hypothesis that the mean difference in weight is equal to zero in the population?

A. Reject both the null and alternative hypotheses

B. Accept both the null and alternative null hypotheses

C. Reject the null hypothesis and accept the alternative hypothesis

D. Accept the null hypothesis and reject the alternative hypothesis

E. It is best not to draw a conclusion about the null and alternative hypotheses from these observations

CHAPTER 4

Univariable Analysis of a Continuous Dependent Variable

CHAPTER SUMMARY

In Chapter 4, we begin investigating the statistical procedures that are actually used to analyze health research data. Up to this point, we have been studying the principles of statistical logic, but using simplified methods. This was to prevent us from being encumbered with too many issues all at once so we could focus on the principles relative to the mean. Beginning in this chapter, that changes.

The most important simplification made in previous chapters was the assumption that the variance of the distribution of data in the population is known. This was so we could assume that chance had an effect on our estimate of the mean, but not on our estimate of the variance. This allowed us to see how we can take chance into account for the estimate of the mean without being concerned about the independent role of chance on the estimate of the variance. Now it is time to

Workbook to Accompany Introduction to Biostatistical Applications in Health Research with Microsoft® Office Excel®, First Edition. Robert P. Hirsch.
© 2016 John Wiley & Sons, Inc. Published 2016 by John Wiley & Sons, Inc.

recognize that there are two, independent, roles of chance when we are calculating confidence intervals or testing hypotheses about a mean.

The standard normal distribution we used in Chapters 2 and 3 appropriately takes chance into account for individuals and for estimates of the mean, but it does nothing about the role of chance in estimating the variance. The standard distribution that takes both of those effects of chance simultaneously is Student's *t* distribution. That distribution takes the role of chance in estimating the mean into account exactly the way the standard normal distribution does. In addition, Student's *t* distribution takes into account the role of chance in estimating the variance. It does this by adding a third parameter called "degrees of freedom."

When a sample is very large, the influence of chance on the estimate of the variance is small. In that circumstance, Student's *t* distribution is almost identical to the standard normal distribution.[1] As the sample becomes smaller, Student's *t* distribution becomes more dispersed (i.e., spread out) than would be the standard normal distribution with the same variance. This increased dispersion is the effect of chance on the estimate of the variance. It causes confidence intervals to be wider and *P*-values to be larger. This reflects our uncertainty about the value of the variance.

The third parameter, degrees of freedom, reflects how much information a sample contains that can be used to estimate the variance. These are the same degrees of freedom we used in Chapter 3 in the denominator of the variance estimate to make it unbiased. For a univariable sample, those degrees of freedom are equal to the sample's size minus one.

Other than the fact that we are using Student's *t* distribution instead of the standard normal distribution, the methods we use to calculate confidence intervals and test hypotheses are the same as in Chapter 3.

GLOSSARY

Continuous Dependent Variable – the variable of primary interest to the researcher which is characterized by having a large number of ordered and evenly-spaced potential values; symbolized by Y.

Degrees of Freedom – a parameter that takes into account the fact that we are estimating the variance of data in the population from the sample's observations. Degrees of freedom in univariable analysis are equal to the sample's size minus one. These degrees of freedom reflect how much information can be used to estimate the variance of data in the population.

Gaussian Family – a collection of standard distributions that are derived from the standard normal distribution.

Paired Sample – two measurements of the same characteristic under different conditions for each individual are made, e.g., a difference in blood pressure

---

[1] In fact, when the sample is infinitely large, Student's *t* and the standard normal distributions are identical.

as measured by the difference between a baseline measurement and a measurement after an intervention. Rarely in practice, a paired sample may involve similar, but not identical individuals for the comparison but, a particular individual must be compared to one and only one other individual.

Paired t Test – a Student's t test performed on data from a paired sample.

Student's t Distribution – a member of the family of standard distributions that are based on the standard normal distribution. Student's t distribution takes into account the influence of chance in estimating the variance. It has as it's parameters a mean (equal to zero), a standard deviation (equal to one), and degrees of freedom (equal to n-1 for a univariable sample).

Variable – represents data in statistical procedures, characterized by type of data it represents (continuous, ordinal, nominal) and its function in the analysis (dependent, independent).

EQUATIONS

$df = n - 1$ degrees of freedom in a univariable sample.

$t = \dfrac{\overline{Y} - \mu_0}{s_{\overline{Y}}}$ conversion of the sample's estimate of the mean to a Student's t value. (see Equation{4.3})

$\mu \triangleq \overline{Y} \pm (t_{\alpha/2} \cdot s_{\overline{Y}})$ two-sided interval estimate for the population's mean in which we have $(1-\alpha)\cdot100\%$ confidence. (see Equation {4.4})

EXAMPLES

Suppose we are interested in the change in weight of persons who stay on a particular diet for three months. To assess this change, each person in a sample of 15 persons was weighed before beginning the diet and again at the end of three months. The values in Table 4.1 are the differences in each person's weight:

4.1. Calculate the sample's estimates of the mean and variance of changes in weight in the population.

The calculation of these point estimates is not influenced by the use of Student's t distribution, thus their calculation is the same as in Exercise 3.1.

$$\mu \triangleq \overline{Y} = \frac{\sum Y_i}{n} = \frac{30}{15} = 2 \text{ lb}$$

$$\sigma^2 \triangleq s^2 = \frac{\sum (Y_i - \overline{Y})^2}{n-1} = \frac{106}{15-1} = 7.57 \text{ lb}^2$$

Table 4.1   **Changes in weight from a sample of 15 persons**

Y	$Y - \bar{Y}$	$(Y - \bar{Y})^2$
4	2	4
2	0	0
3	1	1
−1	−3	9
0	−2	4
10	8	64
2	0	0
−2	−4	16
1	−1	1
1	−1	1
4	2	4
2	0	0
1	−1	1
2	0	0
1	−1	1
TOTAL 30	0	106

4.2. Calculate the sample's estimate of the standard error.

Calculation of the standard error is the same as described in Chapter 3.

$$\sigma_{\bar{Y}} \triangleq s_{\bar{Y}} = \sqrt{\frac{s^2}{n}} = \sqrt{\frac{7.57}{15}} = 0.71 \text{ lb}$$

4.3. Use Excel to estimate the mean, variance, and standard error. How do these compare to the answers in Examples 4.1 and 4.2?

Using the "Descriptive Statistics" analysis tool in "Data Analysis" results in the following output:

Mean	2
Standard Error	0.710465977
Median	2
Mode	2
Standard Deviation	2.751622898
Sample Variance	7.571428571
Kurtosis	4.830051757
Skewness	1.685243752
Range	12
Minimum	-2
Maximum	10
Sum	30
Count	15
Confidence Level(95.0%)	1.52379797

These estimates are the same as the ones calculated in Examples 4.1 *and* 4.2.

4.4. Calculate a 95% confidence interval for the mean change in weight.

Now that we know about Student's t distribution, we use that distribution to calculate confidence intervals. First, we go to Table B.2 *to find the t-value that corresponds to an alpha of 0.05 and 14 degrees of freedom. That t-value is 2.145. Then the confidence interval is:*

$$\mu \overset{\triangle}{=} \overline{Y} \pm (t \cdot s_{\overline{Y}}) = 2 \pm (2.145 \cdot 0.71) = 0.48 \text{ to } 3.52 \text{ lb}$$

4.5. Use Excel to calculate a 95% confidence interval for the mean change in weight. How does this interval compare with the one calculated in Example 4.4?

The width of the 95% confidence interval is part of the output from Excel's "Descriptive Statistics" analysis tool. That output appears in the answer to Example 4.3. *The 95% confidence interval is equal to this value (1.52) added and subtracted from the mean.*

$$2 \pm 1.52 = 0.48 \text{ to } 3.52 \text{ lb}$$

This is the same interval we got in Example 4.4. *Thus, Excel uses Student's t distribution to calculate this confidence interval.*

4.6. What are the most appropriate hypotheses to use in a statistical hypothesis test for these data?

The null hypothesis has to be a specific statement about the population's parameter that makes biologic sense. For a difference between weights, that value is zero. The alternative hypothesis must be a statement of what must be true if the null hypothesis is false. Here, that would be the statement that the difference is not equal to zero.

$$H_0 : \mu = 0 \qquad H_A : \mu \neq 0$$

4.7. Test the appropriate null hypothesis allowing a 5% chance of making a type I error.

Now that we know about Student's t distribution, we use that distribution to test null hypotheses.

$$t = \frac{\overline{Y} - \mu}{s_{\overline{Y}}} = \frac{2 - 0}{0.71} = 2.82$$

From Table B.2, *we find that the critical value of Student's t with 14 degrees of freedom is 2.145. Since the calculated value (2.82) is larger than the critical value*

(2.145), we reject the null hypothesis and, through the process of elimination, accept the alternative hypothesis.

4.8. How can we use Excel to test this null hypothesis?

One way to test this null hypothesis is to use Excel's confidence interval. The null value (zero) is outside of the confidence interval (0.48 to 3.52). Thus, we reject the null hypothesis and accept, through the process of elimination, the alternative hypothesis. The other way is to use Excel's "t.test" function to calculate the P-value. We cannot use this function with this dataset, because it requires that we know the actual weights before and after the intervention, instead of just the differences between those weights.

EXERCISES

4.1. Suppose we take a sample of 36 persons from a particular population and measure their body weights. Then, we give each person a one-month's supply of appetite suppressants. At the end of the month, we weigh each person again and subtract their new weight from their first weight. Suppose we observe a mean difference in weight equal to 10 kg and we estimate the variance of differences in weight in the population to be 900 kg. Which of the following is closest to the interval of values within which we have 95% confidence that the population's mean lies?

    A. −32.2 to 51.8

    B. −0.2 to 20.2

    C. 0.0 to 20.0

    D. 0.2 to 19.8

    E. 2.3 to 17.7

4.2. Suppose we take a sample of 36 persons from a particular population and measure their body weights. Then, we give each person a one-month's supply of appetite suppressants. At the end of the month, we weigh each person again and subtract their new weight from their first weight. Suppose we observe a mean difference in weight equal to 10 kg and that we estimate the variance of differences in weight in the population to be 900 kg^2. Test the null hypothesis that the difference in weight is equal to zero in the population versus the alternative hypothesis that it is not equal to zero. If you allow a 5% risk of making a type I error, which of the following is the best conclusion to draw?

    A. Reject both the null and alternative hypotheses

    B. Accept both the null and alternative hypotheses

    C. Reject the null hypothesis and accept the alternative hypothesis

    D. Accept the null hypothesis and reject the alternative hypothesis

    E. It is best not to draw a conclusion about the null and alternative hypotheses from these observations

4.3. Suppose we were to conduct a study in which 16 persons with hypothyroidism were given two medications in a random order. In this study, we measure TSH after the participants had taken each of the medications for a week. Suppose we estimate the mean difference in TSH levels to be equal to 20 mg/dL and we estimate the standard deviation of differences between TSH levels to be equal to 60 mg/dL. Test the null hypothesis that the mean difference is equal to zero in the population versus the alternative hypothesis that the mean difference is not equal to zero. If you allow a 5% risk of making a type I error, which of the following is the best conclusion to draw?

    A. Reject both the null and alternative hypotheses

    B. Accept both the null and alternative hypotheses

    C. Reject the null hypothesis and accept the alternative hypothesis

    D. Accept the null hypothesis and reject the alternative hypothesis

    E. It is best not to draw a conclusion about the null and alternative hypotheses from these observations

4.4. Suppose we were to conduct a study in which 16 persons with hypothyroidism were given two medications in a random order. In this study, we measure TSH after the participants had taken each of the medications for a week. Suppose we estimate the mean difference in TSH levels to be equal to 20 mg/dL and we estimate the standard deviation of differences between TSH levels to be equal to 60 mg/dL. What is an interval within which we are 95% confident that the mean difference in the population is included?

    A. −88.2 to 147.0

    B. −12.0 to 52.0

    C. −9.4 to 49.4

    D. −5.1 to 36.4

    E. 0.0 to 40.0

4.5. We are interested in the effect of a vegetarian diet on blood urea nitrogen (BUN). To investigate this, we select 12 graduate students who have been eating an omnivorous diet all of their lives. We determine their BUN and ask them to follow a vegetarian diet for 28 days. Then, we measure their BUN again and subtract this second measurement from the initial measurement. Suppose we observe a mean difference of 4 mg/dL and estimate the standard deviation of the differences to be equal to 8 mg/dL. Which of the following is an interval of values within which we can be 95% confident that the population's mean is included?

    A. −1.1 to 9.1

    B. −0.1 to 8.9

C. 0.0 to 8.0

D. 0.6 to 7.4

E. 1.2 to 6.8

4.6. We are interested in the effect of a vegetarian diet on blood urea nitrogen (BUN). To investigate this, we select 12 graduate students who have been eating an omnivorous diet all of their lives. We determine their BUN and ask them to follow a vegetarian diet for 28 days. Then, we measure their BUN again and subtract this second measurement from the initial measurement. Suppose we observe a difference of 4 mg/dL and estimate the standard deviation of the differences equal to 8 mg/dL. Test the null hypothesis that the difference in BUN is equal to zero in the population versus the alternative hypothesis that the difference is not equal to zero. If you allow a 5% chance of making a type I error, which of the following is the best conclusion to draw?

A. Reject both the null and alternative hypotheses

B. Accept both the null and alternative hypotheses

C. Reject the null hypothesis and accept the alternative hypothesis

D. Accept the null hypothesis and reject the alternative hypothesis

E. It is best not to draw a conclusion about the null and alternative hypotheses from these observations

4.7. Patients on a particular treatment often suffer from anemia. To counter this effect, we think that these patients might be helped if they were given folic acid. To evaluate this, we identify 21 patients on the treatment who have been diagnosed with anemia and measure their hematocrit. Then, we give these patients supplemental folic acid for a period of 14 days. Then, we measure their hematocrit again and subtract this second measurement from the initial measurement. Suppose we observe a mean difference between these two hematocrit determinations of −5%. Also suppose that we estimate the standard deviation of differences in hematocrit measurements to be equal to 10%. Based on that information, test the null hypothesis that the mean difference in hematocrit is equal to zero in the population versus the alternative hypothesis that it is not equal to zero. If we were to allow a 5% chance of making a type I error, which of the following would be the best conclusion to draw?

A. Reject both the null and alternative hypotheses

B. Accept both the null and alternative hypotheses

C. Reject the null hypothesis and accept the alternative hypothesis

D. Accept the null hypothesis and reject the alternative hypothesis

E. It is best not to draw a conclusion about the null and alternative hypotheses from these observations

4.8. Patients on a particular treatment often suffer from anemia. To counter this effect, we think that these patients might be helped if they were given folic acid. To evaluate this, we identify 21 patients on the treatment who have been diagnosed with anemia and measure their hematocrit. Then, we give these patients supplemental folic acid for a period of 14 days. Then, we measure their hematocrit again and subtract this second measurement from the initial measurement. Suppose we observe a mean difference between these two hematocrit determinations of −5%. Also suppose we estimate the standard deviation of differences in hematocrit measurements to be equal to 10%. Based on that information, which of the following is an interval of mean differences in hematocrit within which we can be 95% confident that the population's value occurs?

   A. −9.6 to −0.4
   B. −9.6 to 0.4
   C. −0.4 to 9.6
   D. 0.0 to 9.6
   E. 0.4 to 9.6

CHAPTER 5

Univariable Analysis of an Ordinal Dependent Variable

CHAPTER SUMMARY

To perform statistical analysis of ordinal dependent variables, the values of those variables are converted into relative ranks. This is done regardless of whether the variables are from data that naturally occur on an ordinal scale or from continuous data that we wish to convert to an ordinal scale. Such a conversion of continuous data to ranks is done to allow statistical analysis without assuming that the distribution of estimates from all possible samples is a Gaussian distribution.

Conversion of data to ranks can be accomplished by assigning the rank of one to the smallest value, two to the next larger value, and so on. Observations that have the same value, called tied observations, are assigned the mean of the ranks they would have received if they were given separate ranks.

Workbook to Accompany Introduction to Biostatistical Applications in Health Research with Microsoft® Office Excel®, First Edition. Robert P. Hirsch.
© 2016 John Wiley & Sons, Inc. Published 2016 by John Wiley & Sons, Inc.

Estimation of parameters of a population's distribution is not relevant for ordinal dependent variables since no particular distribution is assumed. This lack of assumptions concerning distributions and parameters has led to procedures for ordinal data being referred to as distribution-free or nonparametric procedures. Even so, the median and the interquartile range can be determined from ordinal data and used as estimators of the population's values, even though they are not parameters.[1]

The most common method for performing statistical hypothesis testing on a single ordinal variable is the Wilcoxon signed-rank test. The test statistics for that procedure are the sum of the ranks for the negative differences and the sum of the ranks for the positive differences between paired observations. Unlike for other test statistics, we reject the null hypothesis if the calculated Wilcoxon signed-rank test statistic is equal to or smaller than the value in the table. For a two-tailed test, we calculate both the sum of the negative ranks and the sum of the positive ranks and choose the smaller of the two. A one-tailed test uses either the sum of the positive ranks or the sum of the negative ranks. Which of the two sums is used depends on the alternative hypothesis. Specifically, the appropriate test statistic is the sum that is assumed, according to the alternative hypothesis, to be the smaller of the two sums.

When continuous data are converted to an ordinal scale for statistical analysis, we are able to circumvent certain assumptions about the distribution of estimates derived from all possible samples. We cannot, however, ignore the assumption that dependent variable values are randomly selected from the population.

As a result of this conversion to an ordinal scale, we have the potential for losing statistical power. That is to say, it can become more difficult to reject a false null hypothesis. This loss of statistical power occurs when the assumptions of the statistical procedure for continuous data are not violated, but the data are analyzed as if they were ordinal. The loss of power is usually small and usually has no effect on the conclusions we draw in hypothesis testing.

GLOSSARY

Absolute Value – a value that ignores negative signs, making all values positive.

Median – the physical center of a distribution above and below which are half of the data values.

Nonparametric – statistical procedures for ordinal dependent variables used on continuous dependent variables converted to an ordinal scale. This has the advantage of not assuming a Gaussian sampling distribution.

Relative Ranks – the magnitude of data values in comparison to other data values. The smallest data value gets a rank of one and the highest data value gets

---

[1] Parameters are used in the mathematic description of a distribution. There is no distribution in nonparametric analysis.

a rank equal to the number of data values. Two or more data with the same value are given the average rank.

EQUATIONS

$T_+ = \sum$ Ranks of positive differences   Wilcoxon signed-rank test. (see Equation {5.1})

$T_- = \sum$ Ranks of negative differences   Wilcoxon signed-rank test. (see Equation {5.2})

EXAMPLES

In the examples in Chapter 4, we were interested in the change in weight of 15 persons who stayed on a particular diet for three months. The observations are in Table 5.1.

Table 5.1   Changes in
weight from Table 4.1

Y
5
3
3
−1
0
10
3
−2
1
1
5
2
1
3
1

5.1. Determine point and (95%) interval estimates of the median.

In preparation, we sort the data according to numeric values (Table 5.2).

   The median will be the value above and below which there are half the data values. There are 15 data values, so the median is equal to two. The limits of the interval estimate, we find in Table B.11. *For 15 observations, the limits are the*

third and 13th largest data values. Those values are zero and five. So, we are 95%
confident the median in the population is between zero and five.

Table 5.2   Sorted changes in weight

Y	Sorted
5	−2
3	−1
3	0
−1	1
0	1
10	1
3	1
−2	2
1	3
1	3
5	3
2	4
1	5
3	5
1	10

5.2. Change those data to their absolute values.

To change these values to absolute values, we represent negative one and negative
two with positive one and positive two (Table 5.3).

Table 5.3   Absolute values of changes
in weight for a sample of 15 persons.

Y	$|Y|$
5	5
3	3
3	3
−1	1
0	0
10	10
3	3
−2	2
1	1
1	1
5	5
2	2
1	1
3	3
1	1

5.3. In preparation to use the Wilcoxon Signed-Rank test, rank the absolute values.

Since we are assigning ranks in preparation for the Wilcoxon signed-rank test, we do not rank the value of zero. Among the remaining 14 observations, one is the smallest value. There are five ones, so they are assigned the average of ranks one, two, three, four, and five. Two is the next higher number. There are two twos, so they get the average of the ranks of six and seven. There are four threes, so they are assigned the average of ranks eight, nine, 10, and 11. There are two fives, so they are assigned the average of the ranks of 12 and 13.

Table 5.4   Ranks of absolute values of changes in weight for the Wilcoxon signed-rank test.

Y	|Y|	Rank
5	5	12.5
3	3	9.5
3	3	9.5
−1	1	3
0	–	–
10	10	14
3	3	9.5
−2	2	6.5
1	1	3
1	1	3
5	5	12.5
2	2	6.5
1	1	3
3	3	9.5
1	1	3

5.4. Test the null hypothesis that there is a balance of positive and negative differences in the population versus the alternative that there is not a balance. Allow a 5% chance of making a type I error.

To test the null hypothesis that there is a balance of positive and negative differences we chose the smaller sum of ranks for those observations that were originally positive values and for those observations that were originally negative values. The smaller sum is for the negative values. That sum is $3 + 6.5 = 9.5$. To interpret this sum, we compare it to a critical value from Table B.3. *For 14 (nonzero) observations, the value for an alpha of 0.05 is 21. Since the calculated value (9.5) is smaller than the critical value (21), we reject the null hypothesis and accept, through the process of elimination, the alternative hypothesis. There is a statistically significant imbalance of positive and negative changes in weight.*

EXERCISES

5.1. Patients on a particular treatment often suffer from anemia. To counter this effect, we think that these patients might be helped if they were given folic acid. To evaluate this, we identify 8 patients on the treatment who have been diagnosed with anemia and measure their hematocrit. Then, we give these patients supplemental folic acid for a period of 14 days. Then, we measure their hematocrit again and subtract this second measurement from the initial measurement. Suppose that we observe the following differences: −0.2, 0.5, 0.8, −1.3, −1.4, −5.4, −9.7, −18.2. Create an Excel dataset from those values. Using those data, and without assuming a Gaussian sampling distribution, test the null hypothesis that there is a balance of increases and decreases in hematocrit versus the alternative hypothesis that there is not a balance. If you were to allow a 5% chance of making a type I error, which of the following is the best conclusion to draw?

A. Accept both the null and alternative hypotheses

B. Reject both the null and alternative hypotheses

C. Reject the null hypothesis and accept the alternative hypothesis

D. Accept the null hypothesis and reject the alternative hypothesis

E. It is best not to draw a conclusion about the null and alternative hypotheses from these observations

5.2. Patients on a particular treatment often suffer from anemia. To counter this effect, we think that these patients might be helped if they were given folic acid. To evaluate this, we identify 8 patients on the treatment who have been diagnosed with anemia and measure their hematocrit. Then, we give these patients supplemental folic acid for a period of 14 days. Then, we measure their hematocrit again and subtract this second measurement from the initial measurement. Suppose that we observe the following differences: −0.2, 0.5, 0.8, −1.3, −1.4, −5.4, −9.7, −18.2. Create an Excel dataset from those values. Calculate the median of those values. Which of the following is closest to that median?

A. −4.36

B. −1.35

C. 0

D. 1.35

E. 4.36

5.3. Suppose we are interested in a new treatment for arthritis pain. To evaluate this new treatment, we give it to 100 arthritis patients and ask them to use it for two weeks. At the end of that time, we asked them whether or not their level of pain improved, worsened, or did not change. Suppose that we make the observations in the following table.

Response	Number of Patients
Very much improved	26
Somewhat improved	32
No change	25
Somewhat worse	12
Very much worse	3

Calculate the median of those values. Which of the following is closest to that median?

A. Very much improved

B. Somewhat improved

C. No change

D. Somewhat worse

E. Very much worse

5.4. Suppose we are interested in a new treatment for arthritis pain. To evaluate this new treatment, we give it to 100 arthritis patients and ask them to use it for two weeks. At the end of that time, we asked them whether or not their level of pain improved, worsened, or did not change. Suppose that we make the observations in the following table.

Response	Number of Patients
Very much improved	26
Somewhat improved	32
No change	25
Somewhat worse	12
Very much worse	3

Test the null hypothesis that there was no change in the level of pain versus the alternative hypothesis that there was a change. If you allow a 5% chance of making a type I error, which of the following is the best conclusion to draw?

A. Accept both the null and alternative hypotheses

B. Reject both the null and alternative hypotheses

C. Reject the null hypothesis and accept the alternative hypothesis

D. Accept the null hypothesis and reject the alternative hypothesis

E. It is best not to draw a conclusion about the null and alternative hypotheses from these observations

CHAPTER 6

Univariable Analysis of a Nominal Dependent Variable

CHAPTER SUMMARY

Nominal data can be summarized by probabilities or by rates. Two special types of probabilities we encounter in health research are prevalence and risk. Prevalence of a disease is the probability that an individual chosen at random from a population will have that particular disease. Risk is the probability that a disease-free individual in the population will develop the disease during a specified period of time.

Rates are different from probabilities in that rates contain a measure of time in their denominator. The most commonly used rate in health research is the incidence of disease. Incidence is the number of cases of disease that develop per unit of person-time (e.g., per person-year).

Workbook to Accompany Introduction to Biostatistical Applications in Health Research with Microsoft® Office Excel®, First Edition. Robert P. Hirsch.
© 2016 John Wiley & Sons, Inc. Published 2016 by John Wiley & Sons, Inc.

Estimates of probabilities and rates do not come from Gaussian distributions. Instead, they come from either binomial (for probabilities) or Poisson (for rates) distributions. Interval estimation and hypothesis testing for probabilities and rates are usually accomplished using a normal approximation. A normal approximation means that the distribution of estimates is close to a Gaussian distribution. The justification for using a Gaussian distribution for interval estimation and hypothesis testing on probabilities and rates is that, like means of continuous data, estimates of probabilities and rates from all possible samples tend to come from binomial or Poisson distributions similar to a Gaussian distribution, especially when the sample's sizes are large (this is an application of the central limit theorem).

Standard errors for probabilities and rates are different from standard errors for continuous data. For probabilities, the standard error is a function of the probability itself. For rates, the standard error is a constant. This means that we do not have an independent role of chance in estimating a variance. Since we do not have to make a separate estimate of the variance of data in the population (as we do for continuous data), we do not have to use Student's t distribution to take into account errors in estimating that variance. Rather, normal approximations to the binomial and Poisson distributions use the standard normal distribution.

As with other univariable analyses, statistical hypothesis testing on a single nominal dependent variable is less often of interest than is estimation. A reason for this preference for estimation is the difficulty in formulating an appropriate null hypothesis. When such a null hypothesis can be constructed, however, we can use the normal approximation to the binomial or Poisson distributions to test it. A special case of hypothesis testing for probabilities is the preference test. This is a paired study in which each individual is given a choice of two things and chooses the one she prefers. The null hypothesis is that the probability of preferring one of the choices will be equal to 0.5 (which means there is no preference). The alternative hypothesis is the probability of preferring one of the choices is not equal to 0.5.

GLOSSARY

Actuarial Method – a method for approximating follow-up time when an event occurs between two points of time. This method assumes, on the average, that the events occur in the middle of the period.

Binomial Distribution – the actual sampling distribution for estimates of a probability.

Censored Observations – individuals who have not had the event at the end of the observation period.

Exact Methods – statistical methods that are based on the actual sampling distribution and thus, are not approximations.

Incidence – rate at which new cases of disease occur.

Incident Cases – newly occurring cases of disease.

Normal Approximation – statistical method based on the Gaussian distribution even though the actual sampling distribution is not a Gaussian distribution.

Poisson Distribution – the actual sampling distribution for the numerator of rates.

Prevalence – the proportion of persons who have a disease at a point in time.

Prevalent Cases – cases of disease regardless of when they occurred.

Risk – the proportion of persons who develop a disease over a period of time.

Square Root Transformation – a transformation used in the normal approximation to the Poisson distribution. (see Transformation).

Staggered Admission – when subjects are recruited for a study over a period of time.

Transformation – use of a different mathematic form of an estimate or dependent variable value.

EQUATIONS

$$\theta = \frac{\lambda}{N}$$

parameter of the binominal distribution. (see Equation {6.1})

$$p = \frac{a}{n}$$

sample's estimate of the population's parameter of the binomial distribution. (see Equation {6.2})

$$\mu_p = \theta$$

the mean in a normal approximation to the binomial. (see Equation {6.6})

$$\sigma_p = \sqrt{\frac{\theta \cdot (1 - \theta)}{n}}$$

the standard error in a normal approximation to the binomial distribution. (see Equation {6.7})

$$\lambda \triangleq a$$

parameter and its estimate of the Poisson distribution. (see Equation {6.8})

$$\mu_{\sqrt{a}} = \sqrt{\lambda}$$

the mean in a normal approximation to the Poisson distribution. (see Equation{6.9})

$$\sigma_{\sqrt{a}} = \frac{1}{2}$$

the standard error in the normal approximation to the Poisson distribution. (see Equation {6.10})

$$\theta \triangleq p \pm \left(z_{\alpha/2} \cdot \sqrt{\frac{p \cdot (1 - p)}{n}} \right)$$

confidence interval in the normal approximation to the binomial distribution. (see Equation {6.11})

$$\lambda \triangleq \left(\sqrt{a} \pm \left(z_{\alpha/2} \cdot \tfrac{1}{2} \right) \right)^2$$

confidence interval in the normal approximation to the Poisson distribution. (see Equation {6.13})

$$z = \frac{p - 0.5}{\sqrt{\frac{0.5 \cdot (1 - 0.5)}{n}}}$$

hypothesis test in a preference study. (see Equation {6.15})

EXAMPLES

Suppose we are interested in the occurrence of retinopathy among persons with diabetes. To study this, we randomly select 20 persons from an endocrinology practice who have had adult-onset diabetes for 10 years. Then, we perform an eye examination on these 20 persons. Two of the persons have diabetic retinopathy at this initial examination.[1] The remaining 18 persons are examined for retinopathy annually for 10 years. Table 6.1 shows the results of those examinations:

Table 6.1   Results of 10 annual examinations for retinopathy. Patients with "NE" were not eligible for follow-up, since they had retinopathy at the pre-follow-up examination. "—" indicates a year of follow-up without retinopathy. "X" indicates the presence of retinopathy at the examination at the end of the year.

Patient	Examination									
	1	2	3	4	5	6	7	8	9	10
LE	NE									
AR	—	—	—	—	—	—	X			
NI	—	—	—	—	—	—	—	—	—	—
NG	—	—	—	—	X					
ST	—	—	—	—	—	—	—	—	X	
AT	—	—	—	X						
IS	—	—	—	—	—	—	—	—	—	—
TI	—	—	—	—	—	—	—	—	X	
CS	—	—	—	—	—	—	X			
IS	X									
RE	—	—	—	—	—	X				
AL	NE									
LY	—	—	—	—	—	—	—	—	—	X
FU	—	—	—	—	—	X				
NF	—	—	X							
OR	—	—	—	—	—	—	—	—	—	—
EV	—	—	—	—	—	—	X			
ER	—	—	—	—	—	—	—	—	X	
YO	—	—	—	—	—	—	—	X		
NE	—	—	—	—	—	—	—	—	—	—

6.1. For which patients did we observe prevalent cases of retinopathy?

Patients LE and AL had prevalent cases of retinopathy. We don't know when they developed retinopathy, only that they had retinopathy at the initial examination.

[1] The first examination occurred one year after the initial examination.

6.2. For which patients did we observe incident cases of retinopathy?

We consider patients AR, NG, ST, AT, CS, IS, RE, LY, FU, NF, EV, ER, and YO to have had incident cases of retinopathy. We know that they developed retinopathy in the period between examinations.

6.3. In the entire sample of 20 persons what was the prevalence of retinopathy at the initial examination?

At the initial examination, the only cases are the two prevalent cases.

$$\text{Prevalence} = \frac{\text{cases at point in time}}{\text{persons at point in time}} = \frac{2}{20} = 0.1$$

6.4. In the entire sample of 20 persons what was the prevalence of retinopathy at the final examination?

At the final examination, we have the two prevalent cases plus the 14 incident cases.

$$\text{Prevalence} = \frac{\text{cases at point in time}}{\text{persons at point in time}} = \frac{16}{20} = 0.8$$

6.5. What is the 10-year risk of developing retinopathy?

For calculating the risk, we only include incident cases in the numerator and exclude the two prevalent cases from the denominator. Those prevalent cases were not "at risk" to be incident cases of disease.

$$\text{Risk} = \frac{\text{new cases over period of time}}{\text{noncases at beginning of period of time}} = \frac{14}{18} = 0.78$$

Now, let us think about the incidence of retinopathy. To calculate incidence, we need to calculate the person-time of follow-up. Let us do that for each of the persons in Tables 6.1. For the period during which retinopathy occurred, use the actuarial method to determine person-time.

6.6. Use Table 6.2 to calculate the total person-years of follow-up.

The follow-up times for each subject appear in Table 6.2. There is no follow-up time for the prevalent cases at the beginning of follow-up. Incident cases were assumed to have occurred, on the average, in the middle of the period before they were recognized as cases. Censored observations (those who never developed the disease) contributed 10 years to the follow-up time. The total follow-up time is 124 person-years.

Table 6.2 Table for calculation of person-time of follow-up.

Patient	Examination 1	2	3	4	5	6	7	8	9	10	PT
LE	NE										0
AR	—	—	—	—	—	—	X				6.5
NI	—	—	—	—	—	—	—	—	—	—	10.0
NG	—	—	—	—	X						4.5
ST	—	—	—	—	—	—	—	—	X		8.5
AT	—	—	—	X							3.5
IS	—	—	—	—	—	—	—	—	—	—	10.0
TI	—	—	—	—	—	—	—	—	X		8.5
CS	—	—	—	—	—	—	X				6.5
IS	X										0.5
RE	—	—	—	—	—	X					5.5
AL	NE										0
LY	—	—	—	—	—	—	—	—	—	X	9.5
FU	—	—	—	—	—	X					5.5
NF	—	—	X								2.5
OR	—	—	—	—	—	—	—	—	—	—	10.0
EV	—	—	—	—	—	—	X				6.5
ER	—	—	—	—	—	—	—	—	X		8.5
YO	—	—	—	—	—	—	—	X			7.5
NE	—	—	—	—	—	—	—	—	—	—	10.0

6.7. Calculate the incidence of retinopathy.

The incidence is calculated from the number of incident cases and the person-time of follow-up.

$$\text{Incidence} = \frac{\text{new cases over period of time}}{\text{person-time of follow-up}} = \frac{14}{124} = 0.11 \text{ cases per person-year}$$

6.8. To take chance into account for estimates of prevalence, risk, or incidence we usually calculate a confidence interval rather than test a hypothesis. Why is this the case?

A reason we do not usually test hypotheses about prevalence, risk, and incidence is that there is usually no specific value that has biologic relevance. This means there is no sensible null hypothesis to test.

6.9. For the estimate of the 10-year risk of retinopathy, calculate a 95%, two-sided confidence interval using a normal approximation to the binomial distribution.

$$\text{Risk} = p \pm \left(z_{\alpha/2} \cdot \sqrt{\frac{p \cdot (1-p)}{n}} \right) = 0.78 \pm \left(1.96 \cdot \sqrt{\frac{0.78 \cdot (1-0.78)}{18}} \right)$$

$$= 0.59 \text{ to } 0.97$$

6.10. What is the appropriate interpretation of that confidence interval?

We are 95% confident that the 10-year risk in the population is between 0.59 and 0.97.

6.11. For the estimate of the incidence of retinopathy, calculate a 95%, two-sided confidence interval using a normal approximation to the Poisson distribution.

$$\text{Incidence} = \frac{\left(\sqrt{a} \pm \left(z_{\alpha/2} \cdot \frac{1}{2} \right) \right)^2}{PT} = \frac{\left(\sqrt{14} \pm \left(1.96 \cdot \frac{1}{2} \right) \right)^2}{124}$$

$$= 0.06 \text{ to } 0.18 \text{ cases per person-year}$$

6.12. What is the proper interpretation of that confidence interval?

We are 95% confident that the incidence in the population is between 0.06 and 0.18 cases per person-year.

EXERCISES

6.1.   Suppose we are interested in the risk of peripheral neuropathy among persons with diabetes. To study this relationship, we identify 100 persons with a history of diabetes. At an initial examination, three of those 100 persons were found to have peripheral neuropathy. Five years later, the group was reexamined and 12 additional persons were found to have peripheral neuropathy. Based on that information, which of the following is the prevalence of peripheral neuropathy in this group of 100 patients at the end of the five-year study?

   A. 0.03
   B. 0.07
   C. 0.12
   D. 0.15
   E. 0.17

6.2. Suppose we are interested in the proportion of persons who work for a specific industry who develop chronic obstructive pulmonary disease (COPD). To investigate this relationship, we examine 150 new employees and find that 10 already have COPD. Then, we examine those same 150 persons after they have worked in the industry for 10 years and find 28 new cases of COPD. Which of the following is closest to the point estimate of prevalence of COPD among employees in this industry at the time of the last examination?

   A. 0.19

   B. 0.20

   C. 0.22

   D. 0.25

   E. 0.31

6.3. Suppose we are interested in the proportion of persons who work for a specific industry who develop chronic obstructive pulmonary disease (COPD). To investigate this relationship, we examine 150 new employees and find that 10 already have COPD. Then, we examine those same 150 persons after they have worked in the industry for 10 years and find 28 new cases of COPD. Which of the following is the 10- year risk of developing COPD among employees in this industry?

   A. 0.19

   B. 0.20

   C. 0.22

   D. 0.25

   E. 0.31

6.4. Suppose we are interested in the risk of peripheral neuropathy among persons with diabetes. To study this relationship, we identify 100 persons with a history of diabetes. At an initial examination, three of those 100 persons were found to have peripheral neuropathy. Five years later, the group was reexamined and 12 additional persons were found to have peripheral neuropathy. Based on that information, which of the following is closest to the five-year risk of peripheral neuropathy in this group of patients?

   A. 0.03

   B. 0.07

   C. 0.12

   D. 0.15

   E. 0.17

6.5. Suppose we are interested in the risk of peripheral neuropathy among persons with diabetes. To study this relationship, we identify 100 persons with a history of diabetes. At an initial examination, three of those

100 persons were found to have peripheral neuropathy. Five years later, the group was reexamined and 12 additional persons were found to have peripheral neuropathy. Based on that information, calculate an interval of risk estimates within which we can be 95% confident that the five-year risk of neuropathy in the population occurs. Which of the following is closest to the limits of that interval?

A. 0.02 to 0.22

B. 0.04 to 0.17

C. 0.06 to 0.19

D. 0.08 to 0.17

E. 0.10 to 0.13

6.6. Suppose we are interested in the proportion of persons who work for a specific industry who develop chronic obstructive pulmonary disease (COPD). To investigate this relationship, we examine 150 new employees and find that 10 already have COPD. Then, we examine those same 150 persons after they have worked in the industry for 10 years and find 28 new cases of COPD. Which of the following is closest to the interval estimate for the prevalence of COPD among employees in this industry at the time of the last examination within which we are 95% confident that the population's value is included?

A. 0.18 to 0.32

B. 0.21 to 0.29

C. 0.23 to 0.28

D. 0.24 to 0.26

E. 0.25 to 0.26

6.7. Suppose we are interested in the proportion of persons who work for a specific industry who develop chronic obstructive pulmonary disease (COPD). To investigate this relationship, we examine 150 new employees and find that 10 already have COPD. Then, we examine those same 150 persons after they have worked in the industry for 10 years and find 28 new cases of COPD. Which of the following is closest to the incidence of COPD among employees in this industry?

A. 0.014 per year

B. 0.020 per year

C. 0.022 per year

D. 0.032 per year

E. 0.042 per year

6.8. Suppose we are interested in the risk of peripheral neuropathy among persons with diabetes. To study this relationship, we identify 100 persons with a history of diabetes. At an initial examination, three of those 100 persons were found to have peripheral neuropathy. Five years later, the group was reexamined and 12 additional persons were found to have peripheral neuropathy. Based on that information, which of the following is closest to the incidence of peripheral neuropathy in this group of patients?

A. 0.025 per year

B. 0.026 per year

C. 0.027 per year

D. 0.029 per year

E. 0.032 per year

6.9. Suppose we are interested in the risk of peripheral neuropathy among persons with diabetes. To study this relationship, we identify 100 persons with a history of diabetes. At an initial examination, three of those 100 persons were found to have peripheral neuropathy. Five years later, the group was reexamined and 12 additional persons were found to have peripheral neuropathy. Based on that information, calculate an interval of incidence estimates within which we can be 95% confident that the incidence of neuropathy in the population occurs. Which of the following is closest to the limits of that interval?

A. 0.0 to 0.112 per year

B. 0.001 to 0.056 per year

C. 0.010 to 0.045 per year

D. 0.014 to 0.043 per year

E. 0.008 to 0.048 per year

6.10. Suppose we are interested in the proportion of persons who work for a specific industry who develop chronic obstructive pulmonary disease (COPD). To investigate this relationship, we examine 150 new employees and find that 10 already have COPD. Then, we examine those same 150 persons after they have worked in the industry for 10 years and find 28 new cases of COPD. Which of the following is closest to the interval estimate for the incidence of COPD among employees in this industry within which we are 95% confident that the population's value is included?

A. 0.015 to 0.031 per year

B. 0.017 to 0.039 per year

C. 0.020 to 0.041 per year

D. 0.022 to 0.044 per year

E. 0.025 to 0.030 per year

CHAPTER 7

Bivariable Analysis of a Continuous Dependent Variable

CHAPTER SUMMARY

In this chapter, we encountered bivariable data sets that contain a continuous dependent variable and an independent variable. In previous chapters, we discussed univariable data sets containing only a dependent variable. In those univariable data sets, our interest was in the dependent variable under all conditions. The independent variable in bivariable data sets, in contrast, specifies special conditions that focus our interest on values of the dependent variable. Continuous independent variables allow us to examine how values of the dependent variable are related to each value of the independent variable along a continuum. Nominal independent variables define two groups of values of the dependent variable between which we can compare estimates of parameters.

Workbook to Accompany Introduction to Biostatistical Applications in Health Research with Microsoft® Office Excel®, First Edition. Robert P. Hirsch.
© 2016 John Wiley & Sons, Inc. Published 2016 by John Wiley & Sons, Inc.

The first type of independent variable we examined in this chapter was a continuous independent variable. When we have a continuous dependent variable and a continuous independent variable, we might be interested in estimating dependent variable values that correspond to particular values of the independent variable. When this is our interest, we use linear regression analysis. Alternatively, (or in addition), we might be interested in determining the strength of the association between the variables. With this interest, we use correlation analysis.

Regression analysis can be used to estimate parameters of a straight line that mathematically describe how values of the dependent variable change corresponding to changes in the values of the independent variable. The equation for that straight line includes the intercept (the value of the dependent variable when the independent variable is equal to zero) and the slope (the amount the dependent variable changes for each unit change in the independent variable). The population's intercept is symbolized by α and its estimate from the sample by a. The population's slope is symbolized by β and the sample's estimate by b.

To understand hypothesis testing in regression analysis, it is helpful to understand sources of variation of data represented by the dependent variable. There are three sources of variation, each referred to as a sum of squares or, when divided by its degrees of freedom, as a mean square. The total mean square is the same as the univariable variance of data. The total variation has two components. One component is the variation in values of the dependent variable that is unexplained by the regression line. When this sum of squares is divided by its degrees of freedom, it is called the residual mean square. The other component is the variation in values of the dependent variable that is explained by the regression line. This source of variation is called the regression sum of squares or, when divided by its degrees of freedom (always equal to one for bivariable data sets), it is known as the regression mean square.

The residual mean square is used in estimation of the standard errors used in regression analysis. For hypothesis testing about the population's slope, the standard error is calculated from the residual mean square and the sum of squares of the independent variable.

Hypothesis testing for the slope or intercept uses Student's t distribution. The number of degrees of freedom for that distribution is the number of degrees of freedom used in calculation of the residual mean square $(n-2)$.

In addition to testing specific hypotheses about the slope and intercept in regression analysis, we can test the omnibus hypothesis. The omnibus hypothesis is a statement that knowing values of the independent variable does nothing to improve estimation of values of the dependent variable. It is tested by examining the ratio of the regression mean square and the residual mean square. This ratio is known as the F-ratio.

The F-ratio has a special distribution known as the F distribution. This distribution is related to Student's t distribution, but it has two, instead of one, parameters for degrees of freedom. One parameter for degrees of freedom is associated with the numerator of the F-ratio (always equal to one when we have one independent variable), and the other is associated with the denominator of that ratio (equal to $n - 2$ when we have one independent variable). Table B.4 provides values from the F distribution.

When the null hypothesis that knowing values of the independent variable does nothing to improve estimation of values of the dependent variable is true, we expect the F-ratio to be equal to one, on the average. When that null hypothesis is false, the explained variation in values of the dependent variable (i.e., the regression mean square) will be greater than the unexplained variation (i.e., the residual mean square) in those values. Then, the F-ratio will be greater than one. Thus, tests of hypotheses using the F-ratio are all one-tailed.

When we have only one independent variable, the F-ratio also tests the null hypothesis that the slope of the population's regression line is equal to zero. In fact, the square root of the F-ratio, in this case, is equal to Student's t-value that we would obtain if we tested the null hypothesis that the population's slope is equal to zero.

Alternatively, we might be interested in the way values of the dependent variable vary relative to variation in values of the independent variable. A measure of how two continuous variables vary together is the covariance. The covariance is the sum of the products of the differences between each value of a variable and its mean. Covariance has the desirable property of having a positive value when there is a direct relationship between the variables (as values of the independent variable increase, so do values of the dependent variable) and a negative value when there is an inverse relationship between the variables (as values of the independent variable increase, the values of dependent variables decrease). The magnitude of the covariance reflects the strength of the association between the independent and dependent variables.

The covariance, on the other hand, has a distinct disadvantage in that its magnitude is not only a reflection of the strength of the association between the independent and dependent variables, but is also affected by the scale of measurement. This disadvantage can be overcome by dividing the covariance by the square root of the product of the variances of the data represented by the two variables. The resulting value has a range from -1 to $+1$, with -1 indicating a perfect inverse relationship, $+1$ indicating a perfect direct relationship, and 0 indicating no relationship between the independent and dependent variables. This value is called the correlation coefficient. We symbolize the population's correlation coefficient with ρ (rho) and the sample's estimate of the correlation coefficient with r.

To evaluate the strength of the association between the independent and dependent variables, we square the correlation coefficient. The square of the correlation coefficient (symbolized by R^2) is known as the coefficient of determination. The coefficient of determination (or that coefficient times 100%) indicates the proportion (or percentage) of variation in the dependent variable that is associated with the independent variable.

Interval estimation of the correlation coefficient is not very commonly used in health statistics. More often, we encounter tests of the null hypothesis that the population's correlation coefficient is equal to zero (indicating no association between the variables).

Since estimation of the standard error of the correlation coefficient requires estimation of the variances of the data represented by the independent and dependent variables, hypothesis testing involves conversion of the sample's observations to Student's t scale to take into account the influence of chance on those estimates. The number of degrees of freedom for that conversion is equal to the sample's size minus two. Two is subtracted from the sample's size because two variances of data in the population are estimated from the sample's observations.[1]

For the correlation coefficient to have relevance, values of both the dependent and independent variables must be randomly sampled from the population of interest. The assumption that the dependent variable is randomly sampled from the population is universal to all statistical procedures. Few procedures assume that the independent variable is also randomly sampled (this is referred to as a naturalistic sample). The value of the correlation coefficient, however, can change dramatically as the distribution of the independent variable in the sample changes (such as can occur when a purposive sample is taken in which the distribution of values of the independent variable in the sample is under the control of the investigator).

A nominal independent variable separates values of the dependent variable into two groups. Comparison of values of the dependent variable between those two groups is accomplished by examining the difference between the means in the groups. The standard error for the difference between means is equal to the square root of the sum of the squares of the standard errors of the means in the groups.

In calculating the standard error for the difference between two means, we often assume that the variance of the data in the two groups is the same. This allows us to use all the observations in our sample to estimate a single variance. That estimate of the variance of data is a weighted average of the separate estimates in each group with their degrees of freedom as the weights. The resulting single estimate of the variance of data represented by the dependent variable is known as the pooled variance estimate.

Under the assumption that the variances of data are equal in the two groups, the pooled estimate of the variance is used in place of individual variances when calculating the standard error for the difference between means.

Hypothesis testing for the difference between means uses Student's t distribution. The number of degrees of freedom is equal to the sum of the degrees of freedom in each of the two groups (n-2).

---

[1] Another way to think about this is that it takes a minimum of three points to consider variation from a straight line.

GLOSSARY

Bivariable Variance – variation in the dependent variable after taking the relationship with the independent variable into account.

Coefficient of Determination – proportion (or percent) of the variation in the dependent variable that is associated with (explained by) variation in the independent variable.

Correlation Coefficient – an index (i.e., adjusted for scale of measurement) of the strength of association between two continuous variables that is equal to −1 for a perfect inverse relationship and +1 for a perfect direct association. A value of 0 means there is no association.

Covariance – a number that reflects the strength of the association between two continuous variables as well as the scales of measurement of the variables. A negative covariance indicates an inverse association, while a positive covariance indicates a direct association.

Direct Association – an association between two continuous variables in which values of the dependent variable increase as the values of the independent variable increase.

F-ratio – ratio of two variance estimates. It is interpreted by comparison with the F distribution.

Homoscedasticity – a state in which the variance of the dependent variable is the same regardless of the value of the independent variable.

Intercept – parameter of a linear relationship that reflects the value of the dependent variable when the independent variable is equal to 0.

Inverse Association – an association between two continuous variables in which values of the dependent variable decrease as the values of the independent variable increase.

Least Squares Estimate – an estimate of a parameter that is selected to minimize the squared differences between observed and estimated values of the dependent variable.

Mean Square – the average variation. Equal to a sum of squares divided by degrees of freedom.

Naturalistic Sample – a sample in which both the dependent variable and independent variable values have been selected at random from the population. See Simple Random Sample

Omnibus Null Hypothesis – the hypothesis that states that the independent variable does not help estimate dependent variable values.

Pooled Estimate – combination of two (or more) estimates to result in a single estimate.

Purposive Sample – a sample in which the researcher determines the distribution of independent variable values. See Stratified Sample

R-squared – the coefficient of determination.

Regression Analysis – estimation of the parameters of a linear relationship between the dependent and independent variables.

Regression Mean Square – the average explained variation in dependent variable values.

Residual Mean Square – the average unexplained variation in dependent variable values.

Restricted Sample – a sample taken from a population in which only persons with specific independent variable values are selected.

Scatter plot – a graphic representation of the relationship between two continuous variables. Values of the dependent variable are listed on the vertical axis while values of the independent variable are listed on the horizontal axis.

Simple Random Sample – a sample taken from a population in which persons are selected without regard to independent variable values. See Naturalistic Sample

Slope – parameter of a linear relationship which reflects how much dependent variable values increase for a one-unit increase in the value of the independent variable.

Stratified Sample – a sample taken from a population in which the probability of being selected from the population differs according to independent variable values. See Purposive Sample.

Strength of Association – consistency with which dependent variable values change in a certain direction and with a certain magnitude as values of the independent variable change.

Sum of Cross-products – the amount dependent variable values differ from their mean times the amount independent variable values differ from their mean. Used in estimation of covariance and the slope.

Sum of Squares – the amount of variation of the dependent variable. Compare to mean square.

Total Degrees of Freedom – the amount of information in a sample that can be used to estimate the univariable variation of the dependent variable. The sample's size minus one.

Total Mean Square – the average variation in the dependent variable without regard to the independent variable. The total sum of squares divided by the total degrees of freedom. The univariable estimate of the variance of the dependent variable. (see Univariable Variance)

Total Sum of Squares – the amount of variation of the dependent variable without taking into account the independent variable.

Univariable Variance – the average variation of the dependent variable without taking the independent variable into account. (see Total Mean Square)

Weighted Average – a method for calculating a pooled estimate. Equal to the sum of each estimate multiplied by a weight that determines the contribution of that estimate divided by the sum of the weights.

EQUATIONS

$$\mu_{Y|X} = \alpha + (\beta \cdot X)$$

linear relationship between the dependent and independent variables in the population. (see Equation {7.1})

$$\mu_{Y|X} \triangleq \widehat{Y} = a + (b \cdot X)$$

linear relationship between the dependent and independent variables in the sample. (see Equation {7.2})

$$\alpha \triangleq a = \overline{Y} - (b \cdot \overline{X})$$

estimate of the intercept. (see Equation {7.6})

$$\beta \triangleq b = \frac{\frac{\sum (Y_i - \overline{Y}) \cdot (X_i - \overline{X})}{n-1}}{s_X^2}$$

estimate of the slope. (see Equation {7.4})

$$\sigma_Y^2 \triangleq s_Y^2 = \frac{\sum (Y_i - \overline{Y})^2}{n-1}$$

total mean square. Univariable variance estimate. (see Equation {7.9})

$$\sigma_{Y|X}^2 \triangleq s_{Y|X}^2 = \frac{\sum (Y_i - \widehat{Y})^2}{n-2}$$

residual mean square. (see Equation {7.10})

$$t = \frac{b - \beta}{s_b}$$

test of a null hypothesis about the slope. (see Equation {7.11})

$$t = \frac{a - \alpha}{s_a}$$

test of a null hypothesis about the intercept. (see Equation {7.12})

$$\beta \triangleq b \pm (t_{\alpha/2} \cdot s_b)$$

interval estimate of the slope. (see Equation {7.13})

$$\alpha \triangleq a \pm (t_{\alpha/2} \cdot s_a)$$

interval estimate of the intercept. (see Equation {7.14})

$$\sigma_b \triangleq s_b = \sqrt{\frac{s_{Y|X}^2}{\sum (X_i - \overline{X})^2}}$$

standard error for the estimate of the slope. (see Equation {7.15})

$$F = \frac{\text{Regression Mean Square}}{\text{Residual Mean Square}}$$

F-ratio testing the omnibus null hypothesis. (see Equation {7.17})

$$R^2 = r^2 = \frac{\text{Regression Sum of Squares}}{\text{Total Sum of Squares}}$$

coefficient of determination. (see Equation {7.20})

$$\rho \triangleq r = \frac{\frac{\sum (X - \overline{X}) \cdot (Y - \overline{Y})}{n-1}}{\sqrt{s_Y^2 \cdot s_X^2}}$$

estimate of the correlation coefficient. (see Equation{7.18})

$$\sigma_r \triangleq s_r = \sqrt{\frac{1 - r^2}{n-2}}$$

standard error of the correlation coefficient. (see Equation {7.21})

$$t = \frac{r - \rho_0}{s_r}$$

hypothesis test for the correlation coefficient. (see Equation {7.22})

$$\mu_1 - \mu_2 \triangleq \overline{Y}_1 - \overline{Y}_2$$

comparison of two groups of dependent variable values. (see Equation {7.23})

$$s_{\overline{Y}_1 - \overline{Y}_2} = \sqrt{s_{\overline{Y}_1}^2 + s_{\overline{Y}_2}^2} = \sqrt{\frac{s_1^2}{n_1} + \frac{s_2^2}{n_2}}$$

standard error for the difference between two means not assuming homoscedasticity. (see Equation {7.24})

$$s_{\overline{Y}_1 - \overline{Y}_2} = \sqrt{s_{\overline{Y}_1}^2 + s_{\overline{Y}_2}^2} = \sqrt{\frac{s_{\text{Pooled}}^2}{n_1} + \frac{s_{\text{Pooled}}^2}{n_2}}$$

standard error for the difference between two means assuming homoscedasticity. (see Equation {7.27})

$$\sigma^2 \triangleq s_{\text{Pooled}}^2 = \frac{\sum (n_i - 1) \cdot s_i^2}{\sum (n_i - 1)}$$

pooled estimate of the variance as a weighted average of the group-specific estimates with degrees of freedom as the weights. (see Equation {7.26})

$$t = \frac{(\overline{Y}_1 - \overline{Y}_2) - (\mu_1 - \mu_2)}{s_{\overline{Y}_1 - \overline{Y}_2}}$$

test of a null hypothesis about two means. (see Equation {7.28})

EXAMPLES

Suppose we are interested in the relationship between the basal metabolic rate (BMR) and age in children. To study this relationship, we take a sample of 20 normal children between the ages of 2 and 14 years and measure their BMR. Imagine we observe the results in Table 7.1:

Table 7.1   Basal metabolic rates and age for 20 children

SUBJECT	AGE	BMR
KE	4	52
EP	6	44
ST	8	46
UD	9	47
YI	13	41
NG	7	39
YO	6	41
UR	12	40
EL	10	39
EA	3	56
RN	2	48
IN	8	48
GS	5	44
ST	7	48
AT	2	52
IS	7	44
TI	2	56
CS	4	50
DU	11	39
DE	14	36

7.1 Suppose we want to estimate the mean BMR for children of a specific age. Based on that desire, distinguish between the dependent and independent variables.

We want to estimate BMR so, BMR is represented by the dependent variable. The condition under which we want to estimate BMR is knowing the child's age, making age the independent variable.

7.2 Represent those data graphically as a scatter plot.

We can create a scatter plot in Excel by clicking the Insert tab and selecting a scatter plot. To select your variables, right-click over the graph and choose Select Data. You can label the axes by clicking on the Design tab and clicking on Add Chart Element and selecting Axes Titles.

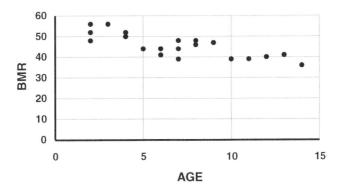

Figure 7.1.   Scatter plot of BMR as a function of age.

7.3 What equation should we use to describe that relationship mathematically?

The regression equation is:

$$\widehat{Y} = a + (b \cdot X)$$

Or more specifically:

$$\widehat{BMR} = a + (b \cdot AGE)$$

7.4 Draw a line on the scatter plot to represent that equation.

To draw a regression line on your scatter plot, right-click on one of the observed values and select Add Trendline. The default will be a straight line.

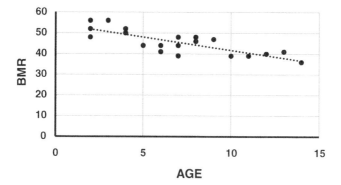

Figure 7.2.   Figure 7.1 with a linear trendline.

7.5 Use the scatter plot to estimate the slope of the regression line.

The slope can be estimated most precisely by looking at the most extreme values of the independent variable. These are ages of 2 and 14 years. At two years, the line appears to coincide with a BMR of 52. At 14 years, the line appears to coincide with a BMR of 36. Thus the slope is approximately equal to:

$$b = \frac{36 - 52}{14 - 2} = -1.33$$

7.6 Use the scatter plot to estimate the intercept of the regression line.

The intercept is the BMR for an age of zero (an extrapolation) which appears to be a BMR of about 55.

Next, let us calculate the estimates of the slope and the intercept. To do that, we need to know the sum of squares for both variables and the sum of cross-products. Those are given in the following table:

Table 7.2   Data from Table 7.1 with calculations for regression analysis

SUBJECT	AGE	BMR	AGE-$\overline{\text{AGE}}$	(AGE-$\overline{\text{AGE}}$)^2	BMR-$\overline{\text{BMR}}$	(BMR-$\overline{\text{BMR}}$)^2	(AGE-$\overline{\text{AGE}}$)•(BMR-$\overline{\text{BMR}}$)
KE	4	52	−3	9	6.5	42.25	−19.5
EP	6	44	−1	1	−1.5	2.25	1.5
ST	8	46	1	1	0.5	0.25	0.5
UD	9	47	2	4	1.5	2.25	3
YI	13	41	6	36	−4.5	20.25	−27
NG	7	39	0	0	−6.5	42.25	0

(continued)

Table 7.2 (*Continued*)

SUBJECT	AGE	BMR	$\overline{\text{AGE}}$- AGE	(AGE- $\overline{\text{AGE}})^2$	BMR- $\overline{\text{BMR}}$	(BMR- $\overline{\text{BMR}})^2$	$(\text{AGE-}\overline{\text{AGE}})$ •(BMR-$\overline{\text{BMR}}$)
YO	6	41	−1	1	−4.5	20.25	4.5
UR	12	40	5	25	−5.5	30.25	−27.5
EL	10	39	3	9	−6.5	42.25	−19.5
EA	3	56	−4	16	10.5	110.25	−42
RN	2	48	−5	25	2.5	6.25	−12.5
IN	8	48	1	1	2.5	6.25	2.5
GS	5	44	−2	4	−1.5	2.25	3
ST	7	48	0	0	2.5	6.25	0
AT	2	52	−5	25	6.5	42.25	−32.5
IS	7	44	0	0	−1.5	2.25	0
TI	2	56	−5	25	10.5	110.25	−52.5
CS	4	50	−3	9	4.5	20.25	−13.5
DU	11	39	4	16	−6.5	42.25	−26
DE	14	36	7	49	−9.5	90.25	−66.5
TOTAL	140	910	0	256	0.0	641.00	−324.0

7.7 Based on those data, what is the sample's estimate of the slope of the regression line?

$$b = \frac{\sum(Y - \overline{Y}) \cdot (X - \overline{X})}{\sum(X - \overline{X})^2} = \frac{-324}{256} = -1.27$$

7.8 Based on those data, what is the sample's estimate of the intercept of the regression line?

$$a = \overline{Y} - (b \cdot \overline{X}) = \frac{910}{20} - \left(-1.27 \cdot \frac{140}{20}\right) = 54.4$$

7.9 How do these values compare with the estimates we made using our scatter plot?

They are very close in value.

7.10 Use the regression equation to estimate the average BMR for 10-year old children in the population.

$$Y = a + (b \cdot X) = 54.4 + (-1.27 \cdot 10) = 41.7$$

7.11 Now use Excel to estimate the slope and the intercept. How do those estimates compare to the ones we calculated by hand?

SUMMARY OUTPUT

Regression Statistics	
Multiple R	0.799826912
R Square	0.639723089
Adjusted R Square	0.619707705
Standard Error	3.58187955
Observations	20

ANOVA

	df	SS	MS	F	Significance F
Regression	1	410.0625	410.0625	31.96156969	2.30924E-05
Residual	18	230.9375	12.82986111		
Total	19	641			

	Coefficients	Standard Error	t Stat	P-value	Lower 95%	Upper 95%
Intercept	54.359375	1.75988882	30.88795973	4.78757E-17	50.66198579	58.05676421
AGE	-1.265625	0.223867472	-5.653456437	2.30924E-05	-1.735953106	-0.795296894

These computed estimates are the same as the calculated estimates except for rounding.

7.12 Use the Excel output to test the null hypothesis that the intercept is equal to zero in the population (versus the alternative that it is not equal to zero) allowing a 5% chance of making a type I error.

The P-value is much less than 0.05 ($4.8x10^{-17}$), so we reject the null hypothesis that the intercept is equal to zero and, through the process of elimination, accept the alternative hypothesis that it is not equal to zero.

7.13 Use that output to test the null hypothesis that the slope is equal to zero in the population (versus the alternative that it is not equal to zero) allowing a 5% chance of making a type I error.

The P-value is much less than 0.05 ($2.3x10^{-5}$), so we reject the null hypothesis that the slope is equal to zero and, through the process of elimination, accept the alternative hypothesis that it is not equal to zero.

7.14 Use that output to test the omnibus null hypothesis that knowing age does not help to estimate BMR (versus the alternative that it does help) allowing a 5% chance of making a type I error.

The P-value is much less than 0.05 ($2.3x10^{-5}$), so we reject the null hypothesis that knowing age does not help estimate BMR and, through the process of elimination, accept the alternative hypothesis that it does help.

7.15 Square the t-value used to test the null hypothesis that the slope is equal to zero. Where in the output can this squared value be found?

The t-value squared is equal to the same value as the F-ratio.

7.16 Another approach to these data would be to estimate the strength of the association between age and BMR. To do that, we can use the R^2 provided as part of the REG procedure output. What is that value?

The R^2 in the regression output is 0.6397.

7.17 How can we interpret that R^2 value?

The R^2 tells us that 63.97% of the observed variation in BMR is associated with (explained by) variation in ages.

7.18 What do we need to assume before we can interpret that R^2 as a reflection of the strength of association in the population?

To conclude that 63.97% is an unbiased estimate of the strength of the association in the population, we need to assume that age has been sampled naturalistically (at random) from the population.

Suppose we have a new diet intended to lower serum cholesterol. To investigate this diet, we measure serum cholesterol before and after the diet and record the difference. Table 7.3 shows the changes in serum cholesterol for men and women.

Table 7.3   Changes in serum cholesterol for men and women.

MEN	WOMEN
29	20
36	14
42	20
48	40
37	11
31	45
41	9
31	42
29	22
35	53
48	
31	
44	
32	

Table 7.3   (*Continued*)

MEN	WOMEN
48	
51	
22	
40	
41	
43	

7.19 Identify the independent and dependent variables.

The dependent variable is the change in cholesterol. That is what we are interested in estimating. The independent variable is gender. That specifies the condition under which we are interested in estimating the change in cholesterol.

Next, we will use Excel to analyze these data assuming homoscedasticity.

t-Test: Two-Sample Assuming Equal Variances

	MEN	WOMEN
Mean	37.95	27.6
Variance	62.26052632	251.3777778
Observations	20	10
Pooled Variance	123.0482143	
Hypothesized Mean Difference	0	
df	28	
t Stat	2.409112397	
P(T<=t) one-tail	0.011407802	
t Critical one-tail	1.701130934	
P(T<=t) two-tail	0.022815604	
t Critical two-tail	2.048407142	

7.20 What is the pooled variance estimate?

The pooled variance estimate is listed in the "Equal Variances" output. It is equal to 123.0482143.

7.21 Test the null hypothesis that the difference in serum cholesterol is equal to zero in the population assuming homoscedasticity. As an alternative hypothesis consider the difference in serum cholesterol. Allow a 5% chance of making a type I error.

The appropriate P-value is "P(T<=) two-tail." That P-value is 0.022816. Since this is less than 0.05, we can reject the null hypothesis that the changes in *cholesterol are the same for men and women and accept, through the process of elimination, the alternative hypothesis that the change in cholesterol is different between the genders.*

7.22 Test the null hypothesis that the difference in serum cholesterol is equal to zero in the population without assuming homoscedasticity. As an alternative hypothesis assume the difference in serum cholesterol is not equal to zero. Allow a 5% chance of making a type I error.

To answer this question, we have to use the output from the "t-Test: Two-Sample Assuming Unequal Variances" analysis tool.

t-Test: Two-Sample Assuming Unequal Variances

	MEN	WOMEN
Mean	37.95	27.6
Variance	62.2605263	251.3777778
Observations	20	10
Hypothesized Mean Difference	0	
df	11	
t Stat	1.947264485	
P(T<=t) one-tail	0.038738838	
t Critical one-tail	1.795884819	
P(T<=t) two-tail	0.077477677	
t Critical two-tail	2.20098516	

The appropriate P-value is "P(T<=) two-tail." That P-value is 0.07748. Since this is greater than 0.05, we fail to reject the null hypothesis that the changes in cholesterol are the same for men and women.

7.23 Which of those two hypothesis tests is more appropriate?

To select the more appropriate result, we can use the "F-Test Two-Sample for Variances" analysis tool.

F-Test Two-Sample for Variances

	MEN	WOMEN
Mean	37.95	27.6
Variance	62.26052632	251.3777778
Observations	20	10
df	19	9
F	0.247677129	
P(F<=f) one-tail	0.00503433	
F Critical one-tail	0.412762801	

The P-value is less than 0.05 (0.005034), so we can reject the null hypothesis that the variances are equal and accept, through the process of elimination, that the variances are not equal in the population. This means that appropriate results are from the "t-Test: Two-Sample Assuming Unequal Variances" analysis tool.

EXERCISES

7.1. Suppose we are interested in the relationship between nerve diameter and nerve conduction velocity. To investigate this relationship, we test 8 nerves of various diameters. These data are in the Excel file EXR7_1.xls on the website accompanying this workbook. Analyze these data as a regression. Based on the results of this analysis, which of the following is the nerve conduction velocity you would expect for a nerve with a diameter of 10 μm?

    A. 6

    B. 8

    C. 15

    D. 32

    E. 48

7.2. Suppose we are interested in the changes in diastolic blood pressure related to age and make the observations in the Excel file called EXR7_2.xls on the website accompanying this workbook. Based on those data, perform a regression analysis. From those results what DBP would we expect, on the average, for persons who are 50 years old?

    A. 76

    B. 80

    C. 83

    D. 86

    E. 89

7.3. Suppose we are interested in the relationship between nerve diameter and nerve conduction velocity. To investigate this relationship, we test 8 nerves of various diameters. These data are in the Excel file EXR7_1.xls on the website accompanying this workbook. Analyze these data as a regression. Based on the results of this analysis, test the null hypothesis that the intercept is equal to zero in the population versus the alternative hypothesis that it is not equal to zero. If you allow a 5% chance of making a type I error, which of the following is the best conclusion to draw?

    A. Reject both the null and alternative hypotheses

    B. Accept both the null and alternative hypotheses

    C. Reject the null hypothesis and accept the alternative hypothesis

    D. Accept the null hypothesis and reject the alternative hypothesis

    E. It is best not to draw a conclusion about the null and alternative hypotheses based on these observations

7.4. Suppose we are interested in the changes in diastolic blood pressure related to age and make the observations in the Excel file EXR7_2.xls on the website accompanying this workbook. Based on those data, perform a regression analysis. Test the null hypothesis that the slope is equal to zero in the population versus the alternative hypothesis that it is not equal to zero. If we allow a 5% chance of making a type I error, which of the following is the best conclusion to draw?

    A. Reject both the null and alternative hypotheses

    B. Accept both the null and alternative hypotheses

    C. Reject the null hypothesis and accept the alternative hypothesis

    D. Accept the null hypothesis and reject the alternative hypothesis

    E. It is best not to draw a conclusion about the null and alternative hypotheses based on these observations

7.5. Suppose we are interested in the relationship between nerve diameter and nerve conduction velocity. To investigate this relationship, we test 8 nerves of various diameters. These data are in the Excel file EXR7_1.xls on the website accompanying this workbook. Analyze these data as a regression. Based on the results of this analysis, test the null hypothesis that knowing nerve diameter does not help estimate nerve conduction velocity versus the alternative hypothesis that it does help. If you allow a 5% chance of making a type I error, which of the following is the best conclusion to draw?

    A. Reject both the null and alternative hypotheses

    B. Accept both the null and alternative hypotheses

    C. Reject the null hypothesis and accept the alternative hypothesis

    D. Accept the null hypothesis and reject the alternative hypothesis

    E. It is best not to draw a conclusion about the null and alternative hypotheses based on these observations

7.6. Suppose we are interested in the changes in diastolic blood pressure related to age and make the observations in the Excel file EXR7_2.xls on the website accompanying this workbook. Based on those data, perform a regression analysis. From the results of the analysis, test the null hypothesis that knowing age does not help estimate diastolic blood pressure versus the alternative hypothesis that it does help. If you allow a 5% chance of making a type I error, which of the following is the best conclusion to draw?

    A. Reject both the null and alternative hypotheses

    B. Accept both the null and alternative hypotheses

    C. Reject the null hypothesis and accept the alternative hypothesis

    D. Accept the null hypothesis and reject the alternative hypothesis

E. It is best not to draw a conclusion about the null and alternative hypotheses based on these observations

7.7. Suppose we are interested in the relationship between nerve diameter and nerve conduction velocity. To investigate this relationship, we test 8 nerves of various diameters. These data are in the Excel file EXR7_1.xls on the website accompanying this workbook. Analyze these data as a regression. Based on the results of that analysis, which of the following is an interval of values within which we are 95% confident that the slope in the population occurs?

    A. −22.0 to 18.8

    B. −2.9 to 6.9

    C. 0.0 to 4.9

    D. 2.9 to 6.9

    E. 22.0 to 18.8

7.8. Suppose we are interested in the changes in diastolic blood pressure related to age and make the observations in the Excel file EXR7_2.xls on the website accompanying this workbook. Based on those data, perform a regression analysis. From the results of the analysis, which of the following is an interval of values within which we are 95% confident that the slope in the population occurs?

    A. 0.42 to 0.57

    B. 1.18 to 9.42

    C. 2.59 to 21.52

    D. 26.35 to 39.2

    E. 50.60 to 60.86

7.9. Suppose we are interested in the relationship between nerve diameter and nerve conduction velocity. To investigate this relationship, we test 8 nerves of various diameters. These data are in the Excel file EXR7_1.xls on the website accompanying this workbook. Analyze these data as a regression. Based on the results of that analysis, which of the following is the proportion of variation in nerve conduction velocity that is associated with differences in nerve diameter?

    A. 0.756

    B. 0.826

    C. 0.890

    D. 0.923

    E. 0.991

7.10. Suppose we are interested in the changes in diastolic blood pressure related to age and make the observations in the Excel file EXR7_2.xls on the website accompanying this workbook. Based on those data, perform a regression analysis. Based on the results of that analysis, which of the following is the proportion of variation in diastolic blood pressure that is associated with differences in age?

A. 0.26

B. 0.44

C. 0.53

D. 0.61

E. 0.78

7.11. Suppose we are interested a diet designed to lower serum cholesterol. When we compare the amount of change in serum cholesterol between men and women we make the observations in the Excel file EXR7_3. Use Excel to test the null hypothesis that the difference of the means of the changes in cholesterol is equal to zero when comparing men and women in the population versus the alternative that it is not equal to zero. If we allow a 5% chance of making a type I error, which of the following is the best conclusion to draw?

A. Reject both the null and alternative hypotheses

B. Accept both the null and alternative hypotheses

C. Reject the null hypothesis and accept the alternative hypothesis

D. Accept the null hypothesis and reject the alternative hypothesis

E. It is best not to draw a conclusion about the null and alternative hypotheses based on these observations

7.12. Suppose we are interested in cholesterol levels among patients who had a myocardial infarction (cases) 14 days ago compared to patients who did not have a myocardial infarction (controls). The Excel file containing those data is EXR7_4. Use those data to compare the means between cases and controls. Test the null hypothesis that the difference of the means of the changes in cholesterol is equal to zero when comparing cases and controls in the population versus the alternative that it is not equal to zero. If we allow a 5% chance of making a type I error, which of the following is the best conclusion to draw?

A. Reject both the null and alternative hypotheses

B. Accept both the null and alternative hypotheses

C. Reject the null hypothesis and accept the alternative hypothesis

D. Accept the null hypothesis and reject the alternative hypothesis

E. It is best not to draw a conclusion about the null and alternative hypotheses based on these observations

7.13. Suppose we are interested a diet designed to lower serum cholesterol. When we compare the amount of change in serum cholesterol between men and women we make the observations in the Excel file EXR7_3. Use Excel to calculate a 95% confidence interval for the difference between the means. Which of the following is closest to that interval?

A. −0.10 to 16.13

B. −0.58 to 15.44

C. −0.12 to 15.08

D. 0.00 to 15.72

E. 0.92 to 15.26

7.14. Suppose we are interested in cholesterol levels among patients who had a myocardial infarction (cases) 14 days ago compared to patients who did not have a myocardial infarction (controls). The Excel file containing those data is EXR7_4. Which of the following is closest to an interval of estimates of the differences of the mean serum cholesterol between cases and controls within which we can be 95% confident that the population's difference occurs?

A. −3.2 to 53.5

B. −1.0 to 44.4

C. 0.0 to 38.2

D. 1.0 to 44.4

E. 3.2 to 53.5

CHAPTER 8

Bivariable Analysis of an Ordinal Dependent Variable

CHAPTER SUMMARY

In Chapter 8, we discover a method of correlation analysis designed for an ordinal dependent variable and an ordinal independent variable. That procedure involves estimation and hypothesis testing for Spearman's correlation coefficient. We learned that there is no method of regression analysis for an ordinal dependent variable.

Spearman's correlation coefficient is calculated from data converted to ranks. Those data can be ordinal or continuous in their natural scale. When a Spearman's correlation coefficient is used to describe the strength of the association between two continuous variables, some of the assumptions of the continuous variable correlation coefficient (Pearson's correlation coefficient) are circumvented. Those assumptions concern the nature of the distributions of the variables. Another assumption of Pearson's correlation coefficient, that the relationship between the

Workbook to Accompany Introduction to Biostatistical Applications in Health Research with Microsoft® Office Excel®, First Edition. Robert P. Hirsch.
© 2016 John Wiley & Sons, Inc. Published 2016 by John Wiley & Sons, Inc.

variables is linear, is also changed. Rather than assume a linear relationship between the variables on their natural (continuous) scale, we assume a linear relationship on an ordinal scale. This is much easier to achieve since it involves only a consistency in direction, not magnitude of dependent variable values.

Preparing to calculate Spearman's correlation coefficient, values of the dependent and independent variables are ranked separately. The easiest way to determine the value of Spearman's correlation coefficient is to use Excel to perform Pearson's correlation analysis on the ranked data. If we wish to test the null hypothesis that the population's Spearman's correlation coefficient is equal to zero, hypothesis testing involves comparison of the sample's estimate of Spearman's correlation coefficient with a value in Table B.5.

When we have an ordinal dependent variable and a nominal independent variable, our interest is in comparing the two groups of dependent variable values defined by the two values of the nominal independent variable. When we considered a continuous dependent variable and a nominal independent variable in Chapter 7, we estimated the difference between means. In contrast, we make no estimates of the difference between the groups when we have an ordinal dependent variable. Therefore, point and interval estimation are not often used when the dependent variable is ordinal.

The method of statistical hypothesis testing we discussed in this chapter for an ordinal dependent variable and a nominal independent variable was the Mann-Whitney U test. We use this procedure to test the null hypothesis that the distribution of the dependent variable is the same in the two groups. The Mann-Whitney U statistic is calculated from the number of observations in each of the two groups and the sum of the ranks in one group (referred to as "group 1"). The choice of group 1 is arbitrary, but that choice will affect the value of the Mann-Whitney U statistic. So, we need to find out what the value of U would have been if we had selected the other group.

When we are considering a two-tailed alternative hypothesis, the appropriate value of the Mann-Whitney U statistic is the larger of U and U'. For a one-tailed hypothesis, the appropriate Mann-Whitney U statistic is calculated by choosing group one to be the group that is hypothesized to have the lower sum of ranks. The appropriate Mann-Whitney U value calculated from the observations in the sample is compared to a value in Table B.6 to complete statistical hypothesis testing.

GLOSSARY

Mann-Whitney Test – a nonparametric method to compare two groups of ordinal dependent variable values. The conclusion of the test is the same as the conclusion of the Wilcoxon Rank-Sum test.

Spearmen's Correlation Coefficient – a nonparametric correlation coefficient that is the same as Pearson's correlation coefficient performed on ranks.

Wilcoxon Rank-Sum Test – a nonparametric method to compare two groups of ordinal dependent variable values. The conclusion of the test is the same as the conclusion of the Mann-Whitney test.

EQUATIONS

$\rho_S \triangleq r_S = 1 - \frac{6 \cdot \sum d_i^2}{n \cdot (n^2-1)}$	a shortcut to calculating Spearman's correlation coefficient that works if there are no tied ranks. (see Equation {8.1})
$U = (n_1 \cdot n_2) + \frac{n_1 \cdot (n_1+1)}{2} - R_1$	Mann-Whitney test statistic. (see Equation{8.2})
$U' = (n_1 \cdot n_2) - U$	alternate Mann-Whitney test statistic. (see Equation {8.3})

EXAMPLES

In the study of changes in serum cholesterol and gender described in Table 7.3, age was also recorded. These data are:

Table 8.1   Changes in serum cholesterol with age for men and women in a sample.

Gender	Age	ChgChol
M	67	29
M	68	36
M	53	42
M	57	48
M	67	37
M	66	31
M	54	41
M	71	31
M	68	29
M	63	35
M	51	31
M	74	48
M	57	32
M	66	44
M	49	48
M	52	51
M	82	22
M	65	40
M	64	41
M	54	43
F	75	20
F	91	14
F	80	20
F	50	40
F	94	11
F	51	45
F	89	9
F	63	42
F	83	22
F	45	53

8.1. Estimate Spearman's correlation coefficient comparing change in cholesterol and age

To begin, we need to represent age and change in cholesterol with their relative ranks. We rank each of those variables using Excel's "RANK.AVG" function.[1]

Gender	Age	ChgChol	RankAge	RankChol
M	67	29	18.5	8.5
M	68	36	20.5	15
M	53	42	7	21.5
M	57	48	10.5	27
M	67	37	18.5	16
M	66	31	16.5	11
M	54	41	8.5	19.5
M	71	31	22	11
M	68	29	20.5	8.5
M	63	35	12.5	14
M	51	31	4.5	11
M	74	48	23	27
M	57	32	10.5	13
M	66	44	16.5	24
M	49	48	2	27
M	52	51	6	29
M	82	22	26	6.5
M	65	40	15	17.5
M	64	41	14	19.5
M	54	43	8.5	23
F	75	20	24	4.5
F	91	14	29	3
F	80	20	25	4.5
F	50	40	3	17.5
F	94	11	30	2
F	51	45	4.5	25
F	89	9	28	1
F	63	42	12.5	21.5
F	83	22	27	6.5
F	45	53	1	30

[1] This is **not** the same as the "RANK" function in earlier version of Excel. In those earlier versions, you can use "SORT" command under the "DATA" tab to order the values and assign ranks manually. With this approach, it is important to sort both columns of data together.

Then, we use Excel's "Correlation" analysis tool on the ranks to estimate Spearman's correlation coefficient.

	RankAge	RankChol
RankAge	1	
RankChol	−0.76196	1

Thus, Spearman's correlation coefficient is −0.76.

8.2. Test the null hypothesis that Spearman's correlation coefficient is equal to zero in the population versus the alternative hypothesis that it is not equal to zero. Allow a 5% chance of making a type I error

To test this null hypothesis, we use Table B.5 *to find the critical value. For n = 30 and α = 0.05, the critical value is 0.362. Since the calculated value (−0.76) is larger (ignoring the minus sign) than the critical value (0.362), we reject the null hypothesis that Spearman's correlation coefficient is equal to zero in the population and accept, through the process of elimination, that it is not equal to zero.*

8.3. Use the Mann-Whitney test to compare changes in serum cholesterol between men and women. Use a two-sided alternative hypothesis and an α of 0.05

To perform the Mann-Whitney test, we need to divide the ranks for changes in cholesterol between men and women from Table 8.1.

MEN	WOMEN	Rank of Men	Rank of Women
29	20	8.5	4.5
36	14	15	3
42	20	21.5	4.5
48	40	27	17.5
37	11	16	2
31	45	11	25
41	9	19.5	1
31	42	11	21.5
29	22	8.5	6.5
35	53	14	30
48		27	115.5
31		11	
44		24	
32		13	
48		27	
51		29	
22		6.5	
40		17.5	
41		19.5	
43		23	
		349.5	

Then, we calculate the Mann-Whitney U considering men as group 1 and U' (the result if we chose women as group 1).

$$U = (n_1 \cdot n_2) + \frac{n_1 \cdot (n_1 + 1)}{2} - R_1 = (20 \cdot 10) + \frac{20 \cdot 21}{2} - 349.5 = 60.5$$
$$U' = (n_1 \cdot n_2) - U = 200 - 60.5 = 139.5$$

With a two-tailed alternative hypothesis, we select the larger of the two as the Mann-Whitney statistic. Here, the larger is U' = 139.5. To interpret that value, we compare it with a critical value. This comes from Table B.6. For 10 and 20 observations and an α of 0.05, the critical value is 145. Since the calculated value (139.5) is less than the critical value (145), we fail to reject the null hypothesis.

EXERCISES

8.1. Suppose we are interested in a diet designed to lower serum cholesterol. When we compare the amount of change in serum cholesterol between men and women we make the observations in the Excel file EXR7_3. Use the Mann-Whitney test to test the null hypothesis that the distribution of the changes in cholesterol is the same for men and women in the population versus the alternative that it is not the same. If we allow a 5% chance of making a type I error, which of the following is the best conclusion to draw?

   A. Reject both the null and alternative hypotheses

   B. Accept both the null and alternative hypotheses

   C. Reject the null hypothesis and accept the alternative hypothesis

   D. Accept the null hypothesis and reject the alternative hypothesis

   E. It is best not to draw a conclusion about the null and alternative hypotheses based on these observations

8.2. Suppose we are interested in birth weights among mothers who have been exposed to second-hand smoke. The observations are in the Excel file EXR8_3. Use Excel to test the null hypothesis that the distribution of birth weights is the same for exposed and unexposed mothers in the population versus the alternative that it is not the same using the Mann-Whitney test. If we allow a 5% chance of making a type I error, which of the following is the best conclusion to draw?

   A. Reject both the null and alternative hypotheses

   B. Accept both the null and alternative hypotheses

   C. Reject the null hypothesis and accept the alternative hypothesis

   D. Accept the null hypothesis and reject the alternative hypothesis

   E. It is best not to draw a conclusion about the null and alternative hypotheses based on these observations

8.3. Suppose that we are interested in the association between the level of exercise each week and the amount of weight change over a four-week period. The Excel file containing these data is EXR8_1. Use Excel to perform a correlation analysis on the ranks of the variables. Which of the following is the estimate of Spearman's correlation coefficient?

   A. −0.427

   B. 0.000

   C. 0.257

   D. 0.427

   E. 1.000

8.4. In a study of serum cholesterol levels among patients who had a myocardial infarction 14 days ago compared to those same patients who had a myocardial infarction two days ago, we find the data in the Excel file EXR8_2. Use Excel to test the null hypothesis that there is no association between the ranks of the measurements at 14 days compared to 2 days versus the alternative that there is an association. If we allow a 5% chance of making a type I error, which of the following is Spearman's correlation coefficient comparing those measurements?

   A. 0.12

   B. 0.25

   C. 0.39

   D. 0.51

   E. 0.69

8.5. Suppose that we are interested in the association between the level of exercise each week and the amount of weight change over a four-week period. The Excel file containing these data is EXR8_1. Test the null hypothesis that Spearman's correlation coefficient comparing variables is equal to zero in the population versus the alternative hypothesis that it is not equal to zero. Which of the following is the best conclusion to draw?

   A. Reject both the null and alternative hypotheses

   B. Accept both the null and alternative hypotheses

   C. Reject the null hypothesis and accept the alternative hypothesis

   D. Accept the null hypothesis and reject the alternative hypothesis

   E. It is best not to draw a conclusion about the null and alternative hypotheses based on these observations

8.6. In a study of serum cholesterol levels among patients who had a myocardial infarction 14 days ago compared to those same patients who had a myocardial infarction two days ago we find the data in the Excel file EXR8_2. Use Excel to test the null hypothesis that there is no association between the ranks of the measurements at 14 days compared to 2 days versus the alternative that there is an association. If we allow a 5% chance of making a type I error, which of the following is the best conclusion to draw?

A. Reject both the null and alternative hypotheses

B. Accept both the null and alternative hypotheses

C. Reject the null hypothesis and accept the alternative hypothesis

D. Accept the null hypothesis and reject the alternative hypothesis

E. It is best not to draw a conclusion about the null and alternative hypotheses based on these observations

CHAPTER 9

Bivariable Analysis of a Nominal Dependent Variable

CHAPTER SUMMARY

Many of the statistical procedures we have examined in this chapter for a nominal dependent variable and one independent variable are very similar to the procedures described in Chapter 7 for bivariable data sets containing a continuous dependent variable. An example is the test for trend which involves estimation of a straight line to describe probabilities as a function of a continuous independent variable.

Testing the omnibus null hypothesis in trend analysis for a nominal dependent variable and a continuous independent variable is similar to the F-test in regression analysis in that hypothesis testing in trend analysis involves examination of a ratio of two estimates of the variation of data represented by the dependent variable. In regression analysis, the F-ratio is calculated by dividing the explained variation (the regression mean square) by the unexplained variation (the residual mean

Workbook to Accompany Introduction to Biostatistical Applications in Health Research with Microsoft® Office Excel®, First Edition. Robert P. Hirsch.
© 2016 John Wiley & Sons, Inc. Published 2016 by John Wiley & Sons, Inc.

square). In trend analysis, we divide the explained variation by the total variation. The reason for this difference between regression analysis and trend analysis is that the total variation of a nominal dependent variable is a function of the point estimates and, therefore, is not subject to separate effects of chance. The ratio in trend analysis has a distribution that is the square of the standard normal distribution. The square of the standard normal distribution is represented by the chi-square distribution with one degree of freedom.

Another parallel between bivariable data sets that contain a continuous dependent variable and those that contain a nominal dependent variable can be seen when the independent variable is nominal. In both cases, the nominal independent variable has the effect of dividing values of the dependent variable into two groups. Similar to comparing means of a continuous dependent variable between two groups, comparison of probabilities between two groups of nominal dependent variable values can be accomplished by examining the difference between those probabilities.

Means are always compared by examining their difference. Estimates of nominal dependent variable values (e.g., probabilities) can be compared by examining their difference or by examining their ratio. A ratio of nominal dependent variable estimates allows us to consider the relative, rather than absolute, distinction between two groups. Differences can be used to compare probabilities or rates. Probabilities and rates can also be compared as ratios.

Another ratio that can be used to compare values of a nominal dependent variable is the odds ratio. The odds ratio is equal to the odds of the event represented by the dependent variable in one group divided by the odds of that event in the other group. Odds are equal to the number of observations in which the event occurred divided by the number of observations in which the event did not occur.

The difference and ratios we have examined thus far assume that two nominal variables are measured for each individual and that only the values of those variables indicate any relationship among the individuals in a set of observations. In another type of dataset for a nominal dependent variable and a nominal independent variable, individuals are paired based on characteristic(s) thought to be associated with values of the dependent variable. In this paired sample, one member of the pair has one value of the nominal independent variable, and the other member of the pair has the other value of the independent variable.

Paired nominal data are arranged in a 2×2 table that is different from the type of 2×2 table used to organize unpaired nominal data. Ratios and differences between probabilities are calculated from a paired 2×2 table using different formulas from those used for an unpaired 2×2 table, but the point estimates are the same regardless of which formula is used. That is not true for odds ratios, which must be estimated using the formula for paired data if the data are paired.

Statistical hypothesis testing for nominal dependent and independent variables uses the same statistical procedures to test the most common null hypothesis about differences as is used to test the most common null hypothesis about ratios. Those null hypotheses are that the difference is equal to zero and that the ratio is equal to one. If one of those null hypotheses is true, then both are true, since they both imply that the nominal dependent variable estimates in the two groups are equal.

Thus, we need only one method of hypothesis testing for probabilities (and odds) and one test for rates. In this chapter, we encountered three alternative methods to test null hypotheses about probabilities. The reason for presenting three alternative methods is that all three are commonly found in health research literature. The first method involves conversion of the difference between probabilities to a standard normal deviate. The standard error for that difference is calculated using a weighted average of the point estimates of the probability of the event in the population.

Another method, known as the chi-square test, is based on the 2×2 table. In this approach, observed frequencies for the four combinations of dependent and independent variable values are compared to what we would expect if the probability of the event were the same for each of the two groups. Calculation of expected values is based on the simplified version of the multiplication rule of probability theory. Then, observed and expected frequencies are compared for each cell of the 2×2 table. Their sum is a chi-square value with one degree of freedom.

The results of those two methods of hypothesis testing are exactly the same with the chi-square value being the square of the standard normal deviate. The popularity of the chi-square test is due, in part, to its ability for expansion to consider more than one dependent and/or independent variable. The chi-square test uses redundant information since only one cell of a 2×2 table needs to be known to determine values in all four cells assuming the marginal frequencies are known.

The third procedure we examined for probabilities and odds uses only one cell of the 2×2 table. This procedure is a slightly different normal approximation, known as the Mantel-Haenszel test.

For statistical hypothesis testing on paired nominal data, we calculate a chi-square statistic using a special method known as McNemar's test.

To test the null hypothesis that the difference between rates is equal to zero or that the ratio of rates is equal to one, we use a method that is similar to the Mantel-Haenszel procedure.

GLOSSARY

2×2 **Table** – a tabular description of frequencies for a nominal dependent variable and a nominal independent variable. The table consists of two rows and two columns delineating four cells.

Cell Frequency – the number of observations that correspond to a particular cell in a 2×2 table.

Chi-Square – a test statistic often used for a nominal dependent variable and (at least) one independent variable.

Concordant Pair – a pair of matched subjects in which both members of the pair have the same outcome.

Contingency Table – an $R \times C$ table in which there are R rows and C columns. 2×2 tables are a special type of contingency table.

Continuity Correction – a correction for a small bias that occurs when representing a discrete distribution with a continuous distribution.

Discordant Pairs – a pair of matched subjects in which each member of the pair has a different outcome.

Dummy Variable – a variable that represents nominal data with numeric, yet qualitative, values. See Indicator Variable.

Fisher's Exact Test – an analysis of a 2×2 table using its actual sampling distribution, rather than an approximation. See hypergeometric distribution.

Hypergeometric Distribution – the actual sampling distribution for 2×2 tables.

Indicator Variable – a variable that represents nominal data with numeric values. See Dummy Variable.

Marginal Frequency – frequencies in a 2×2 table that are sums of rows or columns.

Mantel-Haenszel Test – a chi-square test used to analyze 2×2 tables.

McNemar's Test – a chi-square test for paired 2×2 tables.

Paired 2×2 Table – a 2×2 table that describes the outcomes of pairs, rather than individuals.

Paired Design – a study in which subjects are matched to similar subjects to form pairs.

Test for Trend – strictly speaking, this is an examination of a tendency of the dependent variable to change in a particular direction as the independent variable increases. Most often used to refer to a regression analysis with a nominal dependent variable and a continuous independent variable.

EQUATIONS

$$\theta = \alpha + (\beta \cdot X)$$

population's regression equation for a test for trend. (see Equation {9.1})

$$\chi^2 = \frac{\sum n_i \cdot (\hat{p}_i - \bar{p})^2}{\bar{p} \cdot (1 - \bar{p})} = \frac{\text{Regression Sum of Squares}}{\frac{\text{Total Sum of Squares}}{\text{Total Degrees of Freedom}}}$$

chi-square used in the test of the omnibus null hypothesis in a test for trend. (see Equation {9.4})

$$\theta_1 - \theta_2 \triangleq p_1 - p_2 = \frac{a}{a+b} - \frac{c}{c+d}$$

probability difference. (see Equation {9.5})

$$\frac{\theta_1}{\theta_2} \triangleq \frac{p_1}{p_2} = \frac{\frac{a}{a+b}}{\frac{c}{c+d}}$$

probability ratio. (see Equation {9.6})

$$OR \triangleq \hat{OR} = \frac{\text{Odds of event in Group 1}}{\text{Odds of event in Group 2}} = \frac{\frac{a}{b}}{\frac{c}{d}} = \frac{a \cdot d}{b \cdot c}$$

odds ratio. (see Equation {9.8})

$$\chi^2 = \frac{(a - E(a))^2}{E(a)} + \dots + \frac{(d - E(d))^2}{E(d)}$$

chi-square for a 2×2 table. (see Equation {9.17})

$$\chi^2 = \frac{(|a - E(a)| - 1/2)^2}{E(a)} + \dots + \frac{(|d - E(d)| - 1/2)^2}{E(d)}$$

chi-square for a 2×2 table with continuity correction. (see Equation {9.20})

$$z = \frac{(p_1 - p_2) - (\theta_1 - \theta_2)}{\sqrt{\frac{\bar{\theta} \cdot (1 - \bar{\theta})}{n_1} + \frac{\bar{\theta} \cdot (1 - \bar{\theta})}{n_2}}}$$

standard normal test for a 2×2 table. (see Equation {9.18})

$$\chi^2 = \frac{(a - E(a))^2}{\frac{(a+b)+(c+d)+(a+c)+(b+d)}{n^2 \cdot (n-1)}}$$

Mantel-Haenszel chi-square for a 2×2 table. (see Equation {9.19})

$$OR \triangleq \hat{OR} = \frac{C}{B}$$

odds ratio from paired 2×2 table. (see Equation {9.21})

$$\chi^2 = \frac{(C - B)^2}{C + B}$$

McNemar's chi-square for a paired 2×2 table. (see Equation {9.22})

$$ID \triangleq \hat{ID} = \frac{a}{PT_1} - \frac{b}{PT_2}$$

incidence difference. (see Equation {9.23})

$$IR \triangleq \hat{IR} = \frac{\frac{a}{PT_1}}{\frac{b}{PT_2}}$$

incidence ratio. (see Equation {9.24})

$$\chi^2 = \frac{\left(a - \frac{(a+b) \cdot PT_1}{PT_1 + PT_2}\right)^2}{\frac{(a+b) \cdot PT_1 \cdot PT_2}{(PT_1 + PT_2)^2}}$$

chi-square to compare two incidences. (see Equation {9.25})

EXAMPLES

Suppose we are interested in the dose-response relationship for a medication for control of seizures and we observe the results in Table 9.1.

Table 9.1   Doses of a drug intended to control seizures.

Dose (mg)	n	Seizure
5	10	6
10	10	4
15	10	5
20	10	3
25	10	2

9.1. Have Excel make a scatter plot of these data.

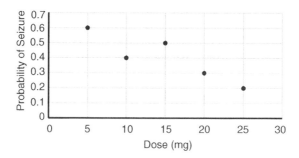

9.2. Test the null hypothesis that occurrence of seizures is not related to dose. Allow a 5% chance of making a type I error.

SUMMARY OUTPUT

Regression Statistics	
Multiple R	0.259807621
R Square	0.0675
Adjusted R Square	0.048072917
Standard Error	0.482830198
Observations	50

ANOVA

	df	SS	MS	F	Significance F
Regression	1	0.81	0.81	3.474530831	0.06844273
Residual	48	11.19	0.233125		
Total	49	12			

	Coefficients	Standard Error	t Stat	P-value	Lower 95%	Upper 95%
Intercept	0.67	0.16013666	4.183926394	0.000121197	0.348023665	0.991976335
Dose	-0.018	0.009656604	-1.864009343	0.06844273	-0.037415904	0.001415904

$$\chi^2 = \cfrac{\dfrac{\text{Regression Sum of Squares}}{\text{Total Sum of Squares}}}{\text{Total Degrees of Freedom}} = \cfrac{\dfrac{0.81}{12}}{49} = 3.3075$$

The critical value is from Table B.7. For $\alpha = 0.05$ and one degree of freedom, the critical value is 3.841. Since the calculated value (3.3075) is less than the critical value (3.841), we fail to reject the null hypothesis.

Now, let us suppose we want to compare the efficacy of a new medication for control of seizures to the standard treatment. To do this, we randomly assign 100 persons to either the new medication or the standard treatment (i.e., 50 to each). Among the persons who were assigned to the new medication, 10 of them had at least one seizure during a two-week period of follow-up. By comparison, 20 of the persons assigned to the standard treatment had at least one seizure during that same period of follow-up.

9.3. Use that information to organize observations in a 2 × 2 table.

Table 9.2   2 × 2 table for two treatments intended to control seizures.

		Seizure		
		Yes	No	
Treatment	New	10	40	50
	Standard	20	30	50
		30	70	100

9.4. From that 2 × 2 table, calculate the two-week risks of seizure for the two treatment groups.

$$\text{Risk}_{\text{New}} = \frac{a}{a+b} = \frac{10}{50} = 0.20$$

$$\text{Risk}_{\text{Stnd}} = \frac{c}{c+d} = \frac{20}{50} = 0.40$$

9.5. Calculate and interpret the risk ratio, risk difference, and odds ratio for the seizure data.

$$\frac{\theta_1}{\theta_2} \triangleq \frac{p_1}{p_2} = \frac{\dfrac{a}{a+b}}{\dfrac{c}{c+d}} = \frac{\dfrac{10}{50}}{\dfrac{20}{50}} = 0.50$$

The risk ratio tells us that persons taking the new medication have half the risk of seizures than do persons taking the standard treatment. The inverse of this ratio (1/0.5 = 2) tells us that persons taking the standard treatment have twice the risk of seizures than do persons taking the new medication.

$$\theta_1 - \theta_2 \triangleq p_1 - p_2 = \frac{a}{a+b} - \frac{c}{c+d} = \frac{10}{50} - \frac{20}{50} = -0.20$$

The risk difference tells us that the risk of seizures is reduced by 0.2 (20%) among persons taking the new medication.

$$OR \triangleq \hat{O}R = \frac{a \cdot d}{b \cdot c} = \frac{10 \cdot 30}{40 \cdot 20} = 0.375$$

The odds ratio tells us that the odds of having a seizure is 0.375 (37.5%) less among persons taking the new medication compared to persons taking the standard treatment. The inverse of this ratio (1/0.375 = 2.67) tells us that persons taking the standard treatment have two and two-thirds the odds of seizures than do persons taking the new medication.

9.6. Use the "2×2 Table Analyzer" BAHR program to analyze this 2×2 table. How do the results compare with your calculations?

When we use Excel to analyze these data, we get the following results:

Observed		Outcome				Expected		Outcome		
		Yes	No					Yes	No	
Group	A	10	40	50		Group	A	15	35	50
	B	20	30	50			B	15	35	50
		30	70	100				30	70	100

Parameter	PE	SE		95% IE	
p(Yes|A)	0.2	0.056569	0.089126	0.310874	
p(Yes|B)	0.4	0.069282	0.264207	0.535793	
Probability Diff	-0.2	0.089443	-0.37531	-0.02469	
Probability Ratio	0.5	0.331662	0.261008	4.945684	
Odds Ratio	0.375	0.456435	0.153287	0.917396	

Test	Chi-Sq	P-value
Pearson's (Uncorrected)	4.761905	0.029096
Pearson's (corrected)	3.857143	0.049535
Mantel-Haenszel	4.714286	0.029913
Fisher's Exact		0.048582

These results are identical to those we got when we calculated these values by hand.

9.7. What are different ways to express the null hypothesis for a 2×2 table that directly address the risk ratio, risk difference, and odds ratio?

The usual null hypotheses we test from 2×2 table data are:

$$H_0 : \frac{\theta_1}{\theta_2} = 1 \qquad H_0 : \theta_1 - \theta_2 = 0 \qquad H_0 : OR = 1$$

All of these null hypotheses are true together or false together.

9.8. Use the Excel output to test the null hypothesis that the risks of seizure are the same in the two treatment groups.

In the output shown above, the P-values (to the far right) are less than 0.05. We do not need that information to answer the question, however. We could look at the confidence intervals and notice that the interval for the probability difference does not include zero and that the intervals for the probability ratio and odds ratio do not include one. All of that information means we can reject the null hypotheses.

One thing we <u>do not</u> want to do is to see if the confidence intervals for the two probabilities overlap. These are univariable confidence intervals. Two univariable confidence intervals are not a substitute for a bivariable hypothesis test!

Now, let us change the underlying frequency of seizures in both treatment groups by making it half of what is was. That would reduce the number of seizures in the group receiving the new medication from 10 to 5 and the number of seizures in the group receiving the standard treatment from 20 to 10.

9.9. Organize these data in a 2 × 2 table

Table 9.3   2 × 2 table for two treatments intended to control seizures with half the underlying frequency of seizures than Table 9.2.

		Seizure		
		Yes	*No*	
Treatment	*New*	*5*	*45*	*50*
	Standard	*10*	*40*	*50*
		15	*85*	*100*

9.10. Use the information in this new 2 × 2 table to calculate the two-week risks of seizure for the two treatment groups.

$$p(\text{SEIZURE}|\text{NEW}) = \frac{\text{Number of Persons on New Treatment with Seizure}}{\text{Total Number on New Treatment}} = \frac{5}{50} = 0.1$$

$$p(\text{SEIZURE}|\text{STANDARD}) = \frac{\text{Number of Persons on Standard Treatment with Seizure}}{\text{Total Number on Standard Treatment}} = \frac{10}{50} = 0.2$$

Both risks are half of what they were in the previous 2 × 2 table.

9.11. Calculate the risk ratio, risk difference, and odds ratio for these new data and compare them to the previous estimates.

$$RR = \frac{p(\text{SEIZURE}|\text{NEW})}{p(\text{SEIZURE}|\text{STANDARD})} = \frac{0.1}{0.2} = 0.5$$

The risk ratio is not affected by the reduction of the underlying frequency of seizures.

$$RD = p(\text{SEIZURE}|\text{NEW}) - p(\text{SEIZURE}|\text{STANDARD}) = 0.1 - 0.2 = -0.1$$

The risk difference is half what it was when it was based on the original frequency of seizures. Thus, the risk difference reflects the underlying frequency of the event.

$$OR = \frac{ad}{bc} = \frac{5\sqrt{40}}{10\sqrt{45}} = 0.44$$

The odds ratio has increased. As the underlying frequency of disease decreases, the odds ratio gets closer in value to the risk ratio.

Another way we could have designed this study would have been to give both treatments to each person at different times. This would be a paired study.

9.12. Suppose the study in Example 9.3 were done as a paired study. Further suppose eight persons had seizures on both treatments. Arrange those results in a paired 2×2 table.

The first step is to use the cell frequencies in the unpaired table as the marginal frequencies in the paired table. Next, put 8 in the upper left-hand cell. Finally, solve for the other cell frequencies by subtraction.

Table 9.4 Paired 2×2 table for two treatments intended to reduce the frequency of seizures.

		Standard		
		SZ+	SZ−	
New	SZ+	*8*	*2*	*10*
	SZ−	*12*	*28*	*40*
		20	*30*	*50*

9.13. Calculate the risk ratio, risk difference, and odds ratio for these new data and compare them to the previous estimates.

The risk ratio and risk difference in the paired table are the same as those estimates in the unpaired table. We can calculate them directly from the paired table by using the marginal frequencies.

$$RR = \frac{p(\text{SEIZURE}|\text{NEW})}{p(\text{SEIZURE}|\text{STANDARD})} = \frac{\dfrac{10}{10+40}}{\dfrac{20}{20+30}} = 0.5$$

$$RD = p(\text{SEIZURE}|\text{NEW}) - p(\text{SEIZURE}|\text{STANDARD}) = \frac{10}{10+40} - \frac{20}{20+30} = -0.2$$

The odds ratio, on the other hand, is different when we have a paired study. It is calculated as:

$$OR = \frac{b}{c} = \frac{2}{12} = 0.17$$

9.14. Test the null hypothesis that the risk of seizure is equal to the same value for both treatments, versus the alternative that they are not equal. If we allow a 5% chance of making a type I error, what should we conclude?

$$\chi^2 = \frac{(b-c)^2}{b+c} = \frac{(12-2)^2}{12+2} = 7.143$$

From Table B.7, we find that the chi-square value that corresponds to 0.05 and one degree of freedom is equal to 3.841. Since the calculated chi-square is larger than the value from the table, we reject the null hypothesis and, through the process of elimination, accept the alternative hypothesis.

9.15. Use the "2 × 2 Table Analyzer" BAHR program to analyze these data. How do the results compare to what we have calculated by hand?

Observed

		Group B		
		Outcome	Not	
Group A	Outcome	8	2	10
	Not	12	28	40
		20	30	50

Parameter	PE	SE	95% IE	
p(Yes|A)	0.2	0.056569	0.089126	0.310874
p(Yes|B)	0.4	0.069282	0.264207	0.535793
Probability Difference	-0.2	0.089443	-0.37531	-0.02469
Probability Ratio	0.5	0.331662	0.261008	0.957826
Odds Ratio	0.166667	-0.67042	0.62018	0.04479

Test	Chi-Sq	*P*
McNemar	7.142857	0.007526

These are the same results we obtained by manual calculation.

EXERCISES

9.1. Suppose we are interested in the number of immunizations necessary to provide protection against hepatitis B infections. To investigate this, we identify a group of persons in a population in which hepatitis B is endemic who had 0, 1, 2, 3, 4, or 5 immunizations and follow them for a period of 10 years. Imagine we observe the data in the Excel file EXR9_1. These data use an indicator of hepatitis B as the dependent variable and the number of immunizations as the independent variable. From that information, estimate the 10-year risk of hepatitis B for a person who had 3 immunizations. Which of the following is closest to that estimate?

A. 0.09

B. 0.12

C. 0.15

D. 0.19

E. 0.24

9.2. In the Framingham Heart Study, 4,658 persons had their body mass index (BMI) calculated and were followed for 32 years to determine how many persons would develop heart disease (HD). Those data are in the Excel file EXR9_2. From those observations, estimate the probability that a person with a BMI of 30 would develop HD during a 32 year period. Which of the following is closest to that estimate?

A. 0.14

B. 0.21

C. 0.29

D. 0.33

E. 0.39

9.3. Suppose we are interested in the number of immunizations necessary to provide protection against hepatitis B infections. To investigate this, we identify a group of persons in a population in which hepatitis B is endemic who had 0, 1, 2, 3, 4, or 5 immunizations and follow them for a period of 10 years. Imagine we observe the data in the Excel file EXR9_1. These data use an indicator of hepatitis B as the dependent variable and the number of immunizations as the independent variable. From that information, test the null hypothesis that the number of immunizations does not help estimate risk versus the alternative hypothesis that it does help. If you allow a 5% chance of making a type I error, which of the following is the best conclusion to draw?

A. Reject both null and alternative hypotheses

B. Accept both null and alternative hypotheses

C. Reject the null hypothesis and accept the alternative hypothesis

D. Accept the null hypothesis and reject the alternative hypothesis

E. It is best not to draw a conclusion about the null and alternative hypotheses from these data

9.4. In the Framingham Heart Study, 4,658 persons had their body mass index (BMI) calculated and were followed for 32 years to determine how many persons would develop heart disease (HD). Those data are in the Excel file EXR9_2. From those observations, test the null hypothesis that knowing

BMI does not help estimate the probability of HD versus the alternative that it does help. If you allow a 5% chance of making a type I error, which of the following is the best conclusion to draw?

A. Reject both null and alternative hypotheses

B. Accept both null and alternative hypotheses

C. Reject the null hypothesis and accept the alternative hypothesis

D. Accept the null hypothesis and reject the alternative hypothesis

E. It is best not to draw a conclusion about the null and alternative hypotheses from these data

9.5. Suppose we are interested in the number of immunizations necessary to provide protection against hepatitis B infections. To investigate this, we identify a group of persons in a population in which hepatitis B is endemic who had 0, 1, 2, 3, 4, or 5 immunizations and follow them for a period of 10 years. Imagine we observe the data in the Excel file EXR9_1. These data use an indicator of hepatitis B as the dependent variable and the number of immunizations as the independent variable. From that information, determine the 10-year risk of hepatitis B for persons who had no immunizations. Which of the following is closest to that risk?

A. 0.119

B. 0.146

C. 0.161

D. 0.261

E. 0.322

9.6. Suppose that we were to conduct a cohort study in which we identified 31 patients who had been diagnosed as having systemic hypertension and another group of 30 patients who had not been diagnosed with hypertension. We followed each of the groups to determine how many developed diabetes. At the end of the follow-up period, there were 25 persons who developed diabetes, 7 of whom did not have hypertension. From that information, which of the following is closest to the estimate of the risk of diabetes among exposed persons?

A. 0.25

B. 0.34

C. 0.42

D. 0.58

E. 0.66

9.7. Suppose that we were to conduct a cohort study in which we identified 31 patients who had been diagnosed as having systemic hypertension and another group of 30 patients who had not been diagnosed with hypertension. We followed each of the groups to determine how many developed diabetes.

At the end of the follow-up period, there were 25 persons who developed diabetes, 7 of whom did not have hypertension. From that information, which of the following is closest to the estimate of the risk ratio comparing the risk of diabetes among exposed persons and among unexposed persons?

A. 0.52

B. 0.61

C. 1.05

D. 2.49

E. 5.14

9.8. Suppose we are interested in the number of immunizations necessary to provide protection against hepatitis B infections. To investigate this, we identify a group of persons in a population in which hepatitis B is endemic who had 0, 1, 2, 3, 4, or 5 immunizations and follow them for a period of 10 years. Imagine we observe the data in the Excel file EXR9_1. From these data, estimate the 10-year risk ratio comparing persons who received no immunization to persons who received at least one immunization. Which of the following is closest to that risk ratio?

A. 0.224

B. 0.581

C. 1.08

D. 1.65

E. 1.80

9.9. Suppose that we were to conduct a cohort study in which we identified 31 patients who had been diagnosed as having systemic hypertension and another group of 30 patients who had not been diagnosed with hypertension. We followed each of the groups to determine how many developed diabetes. At the end of the follow-up period, there were 25 persons who developed diabetes, 7 of whom did not have hypertension. From that information, test the null hypothesis that the risk ratio is equal to one in the population versus the alternative hypothesis that it is not equal to one. If you allow a 5% chance of making a type I error, which of the following is the best conclusion to draw?

A. Reject both null and alternative hypotheses

B. Accept both null and alternative hypotheses

C. Reject the null hypothesis and accept the alternative hypothesis

D. Accept the null hypothesis and reject the alternative hypothesis

E. It is best not to draw a conclusion about the null and alternative hypotheses from these data

9.10. Suppose we are interested in the number of immunizations necessary to provide protection against hepatitis B infections. To investigate this, we identify a group of persons in a population in which hepatitis B is endemic who had 0, 1, 2, 3, 4, or 5 immunizations and follow them for a period of 10 years. Imagine we observe the data in the Excel file EXR9_1. From these data, test the null hypothesis that the risk ratio is equal to one in the population versus the alternative hypothesis that it is not equal to one. If you allow a 5% chance of making a type I error, which of the following is the best conclusion to draw?

A. Reject both null and alternative hypotheses

B. Accept both null and alternative hypotheses

C. Reject the null hypothesis and accept the alternative hypothesis

D. Accept the null hypothesis and reject the alternative hypothesis

E. It is best not to draw a conclusion about the null and alternative hypotheses from these data

CHAPTER 10

Multivariable Analysis of a Continuous Dependent Variable

CHAPTER SUMMARY

When we have a continuous dependent variable and more than one continuous independent variable, we can perform statistical procedures that are extensions of correlation analysis and regression analysis discussed in Chapter 7 for a single independent variable. For more than one independent variable the procedures are called multiple correlation analysis and multiple regression analysis. Both of those procedures examine a linear combination of the independent variables multiplied by their corresponding regression coefficients (slopes).

In analysis of multivariable data sets, we can think about the relationship of the dependent variable to each of the independent variables or about its relationship to the entire collection of independent variables. In multiple regression analysis, both are considered. In multiple correlation analysis, however, only the association

Workbook to Accompany Introduction to Biostatistical Applications in Health Research with Microsoft® Office Excel®, First Edition. Robert P. Hirsch.
© 2016 John Wiley & Sons, Inc. Published 2016 by John Wiley & Sons, Inc.

between the dependent variable and the entire collection of independent variables is considered.

To interpret the multiple correlation coefficient (or, more appropriately, its square, the coefficient of multiple determination) as an estimate of the strength of association in the population from which the sample was drawn, all the independent variables must be from a naturalistic sample. That is to say, their distributions in the sample must be the result of random selection from their distributions in the population.

In multiple regression analysis, we can examine the relationship between the dependent variable and the entire collection of independent variables. The way we do this is by testing the omnibus null hypothesis.

We can also examine each individual independent variable in multiple regression analysis. The relationship between the dependent variable and an individual independent variable in multiple regression analysis, however, is not necessarily the same as the relationship between those variables in bivariable regression analysis (i.e., when we have only one independent variable). The difference is that, in multiple regression analysis, we examine the relationship between an independent variable and the variability in data represented by the dependent variable that is not associated with the other independent variables.

If two or more independent variables share information (i.e., if they are correlated) and, in addition, that shared information is the same as the information they use to estimate values of the dependent variable, we say we have collinearity (for two independent variables) or multicollinearity (for more than two independent variables). Multicollinearity (or collinearity) can make estimation and hypothesis testing for individual regression coefficients difficult. On the other hand, it makes it possible to take into account the confounding effects of one or more independent variables, while examining the relationship between another independent variable and the dependent variable. Multicollinearity is a feature, not only of multiple regression analysis, but of all multivariable procedures.

When we have more than one nominal independent variable, we are able to specify more than two groups of dependent variable values. The means of the dependent variable values for those groups are compared using analysis of variance (ANOVA) procedures. Analysis of variance involves estimating three sources of variation of data represented by the dependent variable. The variation of the dependent variable without regard to independent variable values is called the total sum of squares. The total mean square is equal to the total sum of squares divided by the total degrees of freedom.

The best estimate of the population's variance of data represented by the dependent variable is found by taking a weighted average (with degrees of freedom as the weights) of the estimates of the variance of data within each group of values of the dependent variable. This estimate is called the within mean square.

The within sum of squares is one of two portions of the total sum of squares. The remaining portion describes the variation among the group means. This is called the between sum of squares. The between sum of squares divided by its degrees of freedom (the number of groups minus one) gives us the average variation among group means called the between mean square.

We can test the omnibus null hypothesis that the means of the dependent variable in all the groups specified by independent variable values are equal in the population from which the sample was drawn by comparing the between mean square and the within mean square. This is done by calculating an F-ratio. If the omnibus null hypothesis is true, that ratio should be equal to one, on the average.

In addition to testing the omnibus null hypothesis, it is often of interest to make pairwise comparisons of means of the dependent variable. To do this, we use a posterior test designed to keep the experiment-wise a error rate equal to a specific value (usually 0.05) regardless of how many pairwise comparisons are made. The best procedure to make all possible pairwise comparisons among the means is the Student-Newman-Keuls procedure. The test statistic for this procedure is similar to Student's t statistic in that it is equal to the difference between two means minus the hypothesized difference divided by the standard error for the difference.

It is also similar to Student's t statistic in that the standard error for the difference between two means includes a pooled estimate of the variance of data represented by the dependent variable. In ANOVA, the pooled estimate of the variance of data is the within mean square.

The important difference between Student's t procedure and the Student-Newman-Keuls procedure is that the latter requires a specific order in which pairwise comparisons are made. The first comparison must be between the largest and the smallest means. If and only if we can reject the null hypothesis that those two means are equal in the population can we compare the next less extreme means.

If all the nominal independent variables identify different categories of a single characteristic (e.g., different races), we say we have a one-way ANOVA. If, on the other hand, some of the nominal independent variables specify categories of one characteristic (e.g., race), and other nominal independent variables specify categories of another characteristic (e.g., gender), we say we have a factorial ANOVA.

Factorial ANOVA involves estimation of total, within, and between variations of data represented by the dependent variable just like one-way ANOVA. The difference between factorial and one-way analyses of variance is that, in factorial ANOVA, we consider components (or partitions) of the between variation. Some of these components estimate the variation among the means of the dependent variable corresponding to categories of a particular factor and are called main effects. Other components reflect the consistency of the relationship among categories of one factor for different categories of another factor. This source of variation is called an interaction. Only if there does not seem to be a statistically significant interaction can the main effects be interpreted easily.

It is very common that a dataset contains both continuous and nominal independent variables. The procedure we use to analyze such a dataset is called analysis of covariance (ANCOVA). An ANCOVA can be thought of as a multiple regression in which the nominal independent variables are represented numerically, often with the values zero and one. The numeric representation of a nominal independent variable is called a dummy or an indicator variable. An additional independent variable is created by multiplying an indicator variable by another independent variable. This is called an interaction.

In its simplest form, ANCOVA can be thought of as a method to compare regression equations for the categories specified by values of the nominal independent variables. In that interpretation, the regression coefficient for the indicator variable gives the difference between the intercepts of the regression equations, and the regression coefficient for the interaction gives the difference between the slopes for those regression equations.

Another way to think about ANCOVA is that it is a method used to compare group means while controlling for the confounding effects of a continuous independent variable. This is not really different than the regression interpretation. In fact, all the procedures we have examined for continuous dependent variables can be thought of as regression analyses. This is the principle of the general linear model.

GLOSSARY

ANCOVA – analysis of covariance.

ANOVA – analysis of variance.

Between Mean Square – average variation among groups in ANOVA. Average explained variation.

Bonferroni – method of multiple comparisons that reduces experiment-wise α by reducing the test-wise α.

Coefficient of Partial Determination – the amount R^2 changes when a particular independent variable is removed from the regression equation. See Partial R^2.

Collinear – property of two independent variables in which they are correlated and they share correlated information about the dependent variable.

Confounding – when an independent variable has a biologic association with the dependent variable and is correlated with another independent variable, the second independent variable may appear to be associated with the dependent variable, even though a biologic association does not exist.

Dummy Variable – a numeric variable that represents nominal categories. See Indicator Variable.

Experiment-wise Type I Error – Rejection of, at least one, true null hypothesis among a collection of statistical hypothesis tests.

Factorial ANOVA – an ANOVA in which the independent variables delineate categories of more than one characteristic.

Full Model – a regression equation that includes all of the independent variables. See Reduced Model.

General Linear Model – a principle that recognizes that all methods of analyzing continuous dependent variables can be expressed as regression analyses.

Independent Contribution – the amount an independent variable contributes to estimation of the dependent variable over and above the contributions of all the other independent variables.

Indicator Variable – a numeric variable that represents nominal categories. See Dummy Variable.

Interaction – the circumstance in which the relationship between one variable and the dependent variable is different depending on the value(s) of another independent variable(s).

Main Effect – the relationship between one independent variable and the dependent variable regardless of the value(s) of other independent variable(s).

Multicollinearity – the situation in which several independent variables are collinear.

One-Way ANOVA – an ANOVA in which the independent variables delineate categories of only one characteristic.

Partial R^2 – a measure of the contribution of one independent variable to estimation of dependent variable values over and above the contribution of other independent variables. See Coefficient of Partial Determination.

Posterior Test – pair-wise comparison of means after an ANOVA.

q Distribution – the standard distribution used to interpret the results of Student-Newman-Keuls tests.

Reduced Model – a regression equation that includes some, but not all, independent variables. See Full Model.

Regression Coefficient – the "slope" in multiple regression analysis.

Test-wise Type I Error – Rejection of a true null hypothesis in a single statistical hypothesis test.

Within Mean Square – the average variation within groups of dependent variable values in ANOVA. The unexplained variation of the dependent variable.

EQUATIONS

$$\mu_{Y|X_1\ldots X_k} = \alpha + (\beta_1 \cdot X_1) + \ldots + (\beta_k \cdot X_k)$$

multiple regression equation in the population. (see Equation {10.1})

$$\hat{Y} = a + (b_1 \cdot X_1) + \ldots + (b_k \cdot X_k)$$

multiple regression equation in the sample. (see Equation {10.2})

$$R^2_{\text{Partial}} = R^2_{\text{Full}} - R^2_{\text{Reduced}}$$

coefficient of partial determination. (see Equation {10.4})

$$t_{H_0:\beta_1=0} = \frac{b_1 - \beta_1}{s_{b_1}} = \sqrt{\frac{R^2_{\text{Partial}} \cdot \text{Total SS}}{\text{Residual MS}}}$$

relationship between Student's t-test to test the null hypothesis that a regression coefficient is zero and the partial R^2. (see Equation {10.6})

$$q = \frac{(\overline{Y}_1 - \overline{Y}_2) - (\mu_1 - \mu_2)}{\sqrt{\frac{s^2_{Y|Xs}}{2} \cdot \left(\frac{1}{n_1} + \frac{1}{n_2}\right)}}$$

Student-Newman-Keuls test. (see Equation {10.10}

EXAMPLES

Suppose we are interested in the risk factors for coronary artery disease. To examine those risk factors, we measure the percent stenosis of the coronary artery for 40 patients undergoing angiography for evaluation of coronary artery disease. We also determine their dietary exposure to fat and carbohydrate (measured as percent of total calories), age, diastolic and systolic blood pressure and body mass index (BMI). These data are in the Excel file WBEXP10_1.

Table 10.1   Excel data for risk factors of percent stenosis among a sample of 40 persons.

STENOSIS	FAT	CARBO	DBP	BMI	SBP
61	31	49	62	10	97
53	30	37	60	20	90
44	25	40	62	18	95
63	38	36	60	30	88
63	14	33	70	10	95
60	29	40	68	23	95
51	25	20	63	17	89
65	27	46	75	10	111
65	23	27	88	18	121
70	32	32	97	27	122
55	10	23	71	11	94
60	28	40	97	10	129
56	14	31	91	13	127
65	13	24	102	15	131
72	13	23	95	18	125
55	29	33	70	18	101
67	18	33	73	20	105
71	28	43	91	21	125
58	19	34	78	13	100
52	12	25	61	12	96
70	39	46	109	20	136
74	32	47	81	14	112
67	29	31	105	18	133
69	31	30	70	29	102
67	30	32	93	20	115
69	13	26	87	11	119
83	39	40	92	26	121
57	13	26	68	18	97
68	10	29	105	14	134
67	33	33	75	14	106
80	26	37	104	18	136
92	32	29	120	20	152
69	32	46	78	18	110
65	13	20	104	10	127
67	20	36	88	17	118
67	15	28	102	10	135
75	31	30	107	21	140
72	30	23	92	10	123
87	35	39	127	28	158
66	33	50	62	31	92

When we analyze these data using the "Regression" analysis tool, we obtain the following results:

SUMMARY OUTPUT

Regression Statistics	
Multiple R	0.808259683
R Square	0.653283715
Adjusted R Square	0.613658996
Standard Error	5.965792013
Observations	40

ANOVA

	df	SS	MS	F	Significance F
Regression	4	2347.101398	586.7753495	16.48677246	1.1069E-07
Residual	35	1245.673602	35.59067434		
Total	39	3592.775			

	Coefficients	Standard Error	t Stat	P-value	Lower 95%	Upper 95%
Intercept	20.04491041	6.990523505	2.867440527	0.006963565	5.853393214	34.2364276
FAT	0.20768782	0.16756613	1.239437945	0.223430188	-0.13248951	0.54786515
CARBO	0.089139385	0.153733303	0.579831325	0.565742538	-0.222955812	0.401234582
DBP	0.385323304	0.054865885	7.023003556	3.56815E-08	0.273939636	0.496706971
BMI	0.281648982	0.197711273	1.424546908	0.163144267	-0.11972624	0.683024204

10.1. Use that output to test the null hypothesis that the combination of diastolic blood pressure, dietary carbohydrates, dietary fat, and BMI does not help estimate stenosis

This is the omnibus null hypothesis, so it is tested by the F-ratio (16.49). Since the corresponding P-value (1.1069E-07) is less than 0.05, we reject the omnibus null hypothesis and accept, through the process of elimination, the alternative hypothesis that at least one of the independent variables helps estimate stenosis.

10.2. How much of the variation in stenosis is accounted for by the combination of diastolic blood pressure, dietary carbohydrates, dietary fat, and BMI?

R-Square $* 100\% = 65.33\%$

10.3. What is the estimate of the mean stenosis among persons with a diastolic blood pressure of 90 mmHg, a BMI of 25, and who have 30% of their calories as fat and 50% as carbohydrates?

$$\hat{Y} = a + (b_1 \cdot FAT) + (b_2 \cdot CAR) + (b_3 \cdot DBP) + (b_4 \cdot BMI)$$
$$= 20.04 + (0.21 \cdot 30) + (0.09 \cdot 50) + (0.39 \cdot 90) + (0.28 \cdot 25) = 72.5\%$$

10.4. Which of the risk factors has the strongest association with stenosis when controlling for the other variables?

DBP, since it has the smallest P-value.

Now, let us analyze that same set of data, but without DBP. This is called a "reduced model" since it contains some, but not all, of the independent variables that are included in the original regression (the "full model").

SUMMARY OUTPUT

Regression Statistics	
Multiple R	0.405814478
R Square	0.16468539
Adjusted R Square	0.095075839
Standard Error	9.130378852
Observations	40

ANOVA

	df	SS	MS	F	Significance F
Regression	3	591.6775528	197.2258509	2.365844748	0.087107738
Residual	36	3001.097447	83.36381798		
Total	39	3592.775			

	Coefficients	Standard Error	t Stat	P-value	Lower 95%	Upper 95%
Intercept	57.79311567	6.840547861	8.448609212	4.57879E-10	43.9198415	971.66638975
FAT	0.426279418	0.251989556	1.691655101	0.099352047	-0.084779089	0.937337925
CARBO	-0.172862328	0.228249224	-0.757340263	0.453774821	-0.63577321	0.290048555
BMI	0.191724946	0.301953078	0.634949467	0.52947654	-0.420664279	0.804114171

10.5. How much of the variation in stenosis is accounted for by the combination of dietary carbohydrates, dietary fat, and BMI?

*R-Square * 100% = 16.47%*

Comparing R-square values between the full and reduced models tells us about the contribution of the omitted independent variable(s) to the full model.

10.6. What does the reduced model tell us about the amount of variation in stenosis is accounted for by knowing DBP?

DBP accounts for (65.33% − 16.47% =) 48.86% of the variation in stenosis in the first regression equation (ie, controlling for dietary fat, dietary carbohydrate, and BMI)).

Another way to look at the contribution of some independent variable(s) is to look at a reduced model in which we exclude all of the other independent variables. Let us analyze the data excluding dietary carbohydrates, dietary fat, and BMI and keeping DBP.

SUMMARY OUTPUT

Regression Statistics	
Multiple R	0.717402472
R Square	0.514666307
Adjusted R Square	0.501894368
Standard Error	6.773972556
Observations	40

ANOVA

	df	SS	MS	F	Significance F
Regression	1	1849.080241	1849.080241	40.29664526	1.89878E-07
Residual	38	1743.694759	45.88670419		
Total	39	3592.775			

	Coefficients	Standard Error	t Stat	P-value	Lower 95%	Upper 95%
Intercept	33.33006265	5.245225274	6.354362475	1.86089E-07	22.71165922	43.94846609
DBP	0.383131794	0.060355068	6.347963867	1.89878E-07	0.260949345	0.505314242

10.7. According to that output, how much variation in stenosis is explained by DBP?

*DBP accounts for 51.47% (R-square * 100%) of the variation in stenosis if it is the only independent variable in the model.*

10.8. How does this compare to the amount of variation in stenosis explained by DBP in Example 10.6?

In Example 10.6, we found that DBP accounts for 48.86% of the variation in stenosis over and above that which is explained by the combination of dietary carbohydrates, dietary fat, and BMI. In Example 10.7, we found that DBP accounts for 51.47% of the variation in stenosis. The difference between these values is 2.61%.

10.9. What does this difference tell us?

The 2.61% is the variation in stenosis that is shared by DBP and the combination of dietary carbohydrates, dietary fat, and BMI over and above the variation explained by DBP alone. It tells us about the magnitude of collinearity (in this case, small).

Now, let us suppose we are not sure whether we should use DBP or SBP (systolic blood pressure) to represent blood pressure in our regression analysis, so we include both. Let us analyze the data doing that.

SUMMARY OUTPUT

Regression Statistics	
Multiple R	0.814025898
R Square	0.662638163
Adjusted R Square	0.613026128
Standard Error	5.970676316
Observations	40

ANOVA

	df	SS	MS	F	Significance F
Regression	5	2380.709827	476.1419654	13.35639963	3.13315E-07
Residual	34	1212.065173	35.64897567		
Total	39	3592.775			

	Coefficients	Standard Error	t Stat	P-value	Lower 95%	Upper 95%
Intercept	13.0481685	10.0436123	1.299150954	0.202633317	-7.362907443	33.45924445
FAT	0.212367931	0.167772575	1.265808381	0.214186932	-0.128586963	0.553322825
CARBO	0.047128229	0.159827217	0.29486986	0.769886358	-0.277679755	0.371936213
BMI	0.307367405	0.199638116	1.539622852	0.132908505	-0.098346059	0.713080869
SBP	0.266620314	0.27459502	0.970958303	0.33842622	-0.291423907	0.824664536
DBP	0.116969313	0.281782549	0.415104888	0.680673016	-0.455681725	0.689620352

10.10. Using that output, test the null hypothesis that the combination of diastolic blood pressure, systolic blood pressure, dietary carbohydrates, dietary fat, and BMI does not help estimate stenosis

This is the omnibus null hypothesis, so it is tested by the F-ratio (13.36). Since the corresponding P-value (3.13315E-07) is less than 0.05, we reject the omnibus null hypothesis.

10.11. Now, test the null hypotheses that each of the regression coefficients is equal to zero in the population. What did we find?

None of those null hypotheses is rejected.

10.12. What does that imply?

Since we can reject the omnibus null hypothesis, we conclude that one or more of the independent variables is helping to estimate dependent variable values, but we cannot tell which they are, because none of the independent variables are "significant." The only explanation for this observation is that two or more independent variables are sharing most of the information that they use to estimate dependent variable values. In other words, there is substantial multi collinearity.

For independent variables to be collinear, they must (1) share information and (2) have some of that shared information used to estimate dependent variable values.

10.13. Based on that information, what would we expect to see if we performed a correlation analysis between SBP and DBP?

They should be correlated.

Next, we will perform a bivariable correlation analysis between these two independent variables.

	SBP	*DBP*
SBP	1	
DBP	0.979442	1

10.14. Did we see what we expected to see?

Yes. SBP and DBP are highly correlated (r = 0.979442).

To see if the shared information is used to estimate dependent variable values, we can examine the relationship between the collinear variables and the dependent variable one at a time. The first analysis we did shows that DBP, in the absence of SBP, is a statistically significant estimator of stenosis.

10.15. What would we expect to see if we performed a regression analysis including systolic blood pressure, dietary carbohydrates, dietary fat, and BMI, but excluding DBP?

SBP should be a significant estimator of stenosis. This is because, to be collinear, both (or more) of the collinear independent variables must be estimators of the dependent variable.

If we do that analysis, we observe the following results:

SUMMARY OUTPUT

Regression Statistics	
Multiple R	0.812975038
R Square	0.660928413
Adjusted R Square	0.622177374
Standard Error	5.899655974
Observations	40

ANOVA

	df	SS	MS	F	Significance F
Regression	4	2374.567078	593.6417696	17.05576	7.57365E-08
Residual	35	1218.207922	34.80594062		
Total	39	3592.775			

	Coefficients	Standard Error	t Stat	P-value	Lower 95%	Upper 95%
Intercept	10.54940181	7.944176432	1.32794153	0.19279309	-5.578133751	26.67693736
FAT	0.216850227	0.165433237	1.310802051	0.198460732	-0.1189971	0.552697553
CARBO	0.026491688	0.150092011	0.176502985	0.860916177	-0.278211294	0.33119467
BMI	0.317115183	0.195894033	1.618809814	0.114465759	-0.080570846	0.714801212
SBP	0.378420851	0.052873679	7.157074358	2.39832E-08	0.271081576	0.485760125

10.16. Did we see what we expected?

Yes. SBP is a significant estimator of stenosis.

Suppose we are interested in comparing three treatments for coronary heart disease: (1) bypass surgery, (2) stent implantation, and (3) balloon angioplasty; and two drugs. To do this, we randomly assign 30 persons to one of the three treatment groups (10 per group). Six months after treatment, we measure the percent stenosis of the treated artery. Imagine we observe the results in Table 10.2 (WBEXP10_17).

Table 10.2 Excel dataset for drugs and procedures effect on percent stenosis.

BYPASS	STENT	ANGIO
28	30	48
15	45	35
22	24	30
17	33	35
32	30	60
40	55	55
36	38	44
44	42	62
29	54	50
18	38	48

The null hypothesis usually of interest when we have data such as these is that the means in the groups are all equal to the same value in the population. If this null hypothesis is true, then we would expect to see, in the long run, that the average variation among the means is equal to the average variation among the observations. The average variation among the observations is the within mean square. The average variation among the means is equal to the between sum of squares divided by the number of independent variables needed to separate the data into groups (equal to the number of groups minus one). This is called the between mean square.

If the omnibus null hypothesis (that the means are equal) is true, then the two mean squares will be equal (on the average). We compare mean squares as an *F*-ratio, just as we do in regression analysis.

10.17. Analyze this set of data using the "ANOVA: Single Factor" analysis tool. What conclusion do we draw about the omnibus null hypothesis?

Anova: Single Factor

SUMMARY

Groups	Count	Sum	Average	Variance
BYPASS	10	281	28.1	100.7666667
STENT	10	389	38.9	105.6555556
ANGIO	10	467	46.7	117.1222222

ANOVA

Source of Variation	SS	df	MS	F	P-value	F crit
Between Groups	1744.8	2	872.4	8.089151413	0.001767363	3.354130829
Within Groups	2911.9	27	107.8481481			
Total	4656.7	29				

The P-value for the omnibus null hypothesis is 7.57365E-08. Since this is less than 0.05, we reject the omnibus null hypothesis.

Rejection of a null hypothesis allows us to accept, through the process of elimination, the alternative hypothesis

10.18. What does the alternative hypothesis tell us about the means of the three treatment groups?

That there is at least one difference among the means.

To distinguish among those possibilities, we need to make pair-wise comparisons of the means in a "posterior" test. One of these is the Student-Newman-Keuls test.

10.19. Use the Student-Newman-Keuls test to compare the means. What do these results tell us about the relationships among the means?

To calculate q-values manually, we begin by arranging the means in order of magnitude

Table 10.6   Means of percent stenosis arranged in order of numeric magnitude.

BYPASS	*STENT*	*ANGIO*
28.1	*38.9*	*46.7*

Then, we compare the most extreme means.

$$q = \frac{(\overline{Y}_B - \overline{Y}_A) - \mu_B - \mu_A}{\sqrt{\frac{s_{Y|Xs}^2}{2}\left(\frac{1}{n_B} + \frac{1}{n_A}\right)}} = \frac{(28.1 - 46.7) - 0}{\sqrt{\frac{107.848}{2}\left(\frac{1}{10} + \frac{1}{10}\right)}} = \frac{-18.6}{3.284} = -5.664$$

We compare that calculated value to the critical value from Table B.8. That critical value is 3.486. Since the absolute value of the calculated value is greater than the critical value, we reject the null hypothesis that these two means are equal to the same value. Because that null hypothesis is rejected, we can compare less extreme means.

$$q = \frac{(\overline{Y}_B - \overline{Y}_S) - \mu_B - \mu_S}{\sqrt{\frac{s_{Y|Xs}^2}{2}\left(\frac{1}{n_B} + \frac{1}{n_S}\right)}} = \frac{(28.1 - 38.9) - 0}{\sqrt{\frac{107.848}{2}\left(\frac{1}{10} + \frac{1}{10}\right)}} = \frac{-10.8}{3.284} = -3.289$$

$$q = \frac{(\overline{Y}_S - \overline{Y}_A) - \mu_S - \mu_A}{\sqrt{\frac{s_{Y|Xs}^2}{2}\left(\frac{1}{n_S} + \frac{1}{n_A}\right)}} = \frac{(38.9 - 46.7) - 0}{\sqrt{\frac{107.848}{2}\left(\frac{1}{10} + \frac{1}{10}\right)}} = \frac{-7.8}{3.284} = -2.375$$

The critical value for these comparisons is 2.888. The absolute calculated value for BYPASS vs STENT is greater than the critical value, but the absolute calculated value for STENT vs ANGIO is less than the critical value. BYPASS is significantly different from ANGIO and STENT, but ANGIO and STENT are not significantly different from each other.

Now, let us recognize that we have two drugs (Drug 1 and Drug 2) that are intended to reduce the rate of re-stenosis post-treatment. Suppose we randomly assign half the persons in each of the three treatment groups to one of those drugs (i.e., five in each group assigned one of the drugs).

	BYPASS	STENT	ANGIO
DRUG1	28	30	48
DRUG1	15	45	35
DRUG1	22	24	30
DRUG1	17	33	35
DRUG1	32	30	60
DRUG2	40	55	55
DRUG2	36	38	44
DRUG2	44	42	62
DRUG2	29	54	50
DRUG2	18	38	48

Now, we have six groups of dependent variable values instead of three. More importantly, we have two factors (i.e., characteristics) that are used to create those groups. One of these is treatment group and the other is drug group. As before, treatment group has three categories: BYPASS, STENT, and ANGIO. Drug group has two categories: DRUG 1 and DRUG 2. Both factors together account for $3 \times 2 = 6$ groups of dependent variable values.

When the groups of dependent variable values are specified by more than one characteristic, we can separate the variation between the groups into main effects and interactions. The main effects address the variation between groups specified by just one factor. Interactions address the consistency of the main effects. Use the "ANOVA: Two-Factor With Replication" analysis tool to consider both treatment and drug.

When we have only one characteristic that divides the dependent variable into groups (i.e., one-way ANOVA), this is the only null hypothesis we can test. When we have more than one factor, we can test null hypotheses about the main effects and interactions.

10.20. At which of those results should we look first? Why?

We should first look at the interaction using "ANOVA: Two Factor With Replication" analysis tool. If it is statistically significant, we will not interpret the main effects.

10.21. Interpret the main effects and interactions in the output from Excel

The interaction is not significant, so we can look at the main effects. Both main effects have P-values less than 0.05.

There are only two categories of drug, so rejection of the null hypothesis for that main effect leads to acceptance of the alternative hypothesis that those two means are not equal. Rejection of the null hypothesis for the main effect of treatment group, however, does not tell us which means are different from which other means. Just like in one-way ANOVA, we need to perform a posterior test to see which means are significantly different.

For this set of data, we concluded there was no interaction between treatment group and drug. If we look at the means for those six groups (in the table), we see that, regardless of which treatment group to which people were assigned, those who received Drug 1 had a mean percent stenosis that was about 11% greater than those who received Drug 2. Also, the highest percent stenosis was seen among persons who had angioplasty and the lowest percent stenosis was seen among persons who had bypass surgery, regardless of which drug they received. This is what we imply when we say there is not an interaction between factors; the relationship between categories of one factor is not influenced by categories of another factor.

To see what interaction looks like, let us analyze a new dataset (WBEXP10_22).

Table 10.3 Excel dataset for drugs and procedures effect on percent stenosis with interaction.

	BYPASS	STENT	ANGIO
DRUG1	40	30	48
DRUG1	36	45	35
DRUG1	44	24	30
DRUG1	29	33	35
DRUG1	18	30	60
DRUG2	28	55	55
DRUG2	15	38	44
DRUG2	22	42	62
DRUG2	17	54	50
DRUG2	32	38	48

Let use the "ANOVA: Two-Factor With Replication" analysis tool to analyze the new dataset.

Anova: Two-Factor With Replication

SUMMARY	BYPASS	STENT	ANGIO	Total
DRUG1				
Count	5	5	5	15
Sum	167	162	208	537
Average	33.4	32.4	41.6	35.8
Variance	104.8	60.3	150.3	108.3142857
DRUG2				
Count	5	5	5	15
Sum	114	227	259	600
Average	22.8	45.4	51.8	40
Variance	51.7	71.8	48.2	214.8571429
Total				
Count	10	10	10	
Sum	281	389	467	
Average	28.1	38.9	46.7	
Variance	100.7666667	105.6555556	117.1222222	

ANOVA

Source of Variation	SS	d f	MS	F	P-value	F crit
Sample	132.3	1	132.3	1.629644837	0.213966837	4.259677273
Columns	1744.8	2	872.4	10.74604804	0.00046484	3.402826105
Interaction	831.2	2	415.6	5.119277356	0.014071805	3.402826105
Within	1948.4	24	81.18333333			
Total	4656.7	29				

10.22. Interpret the main effects and interactions in the output from the "ANOVA: Two-Factor With Replication" analysis tool

Now, the interaction is statistically significant, so we cannot interpret the main effects.

Next, let us represent these in data in an ANCOVA. To do that, we need to add the indicator variables for the treatment groups. We could use either of the indicators that we discussed in the text. The only rule is that the numeric values need to be confined to zero, plus one, and, perhaps, minus one. We select from these numeric values since they have qualitative, rather than quantitative natures. For now, let us suppose we are interested in comparing the mean percent stenosis estimate for persons who received a stent to the mean percent stenosis estimate for persons who had bypass surgery and to the mean percent stenosis estimate for persons who had angioplasty.

10.23. How should we define the indicator variables to facilitate those comparisons?

When we want to compare all groups to one specific group, we need to use 0, 1 indicator variables with the comparison group assigned zero for all the indicator variables.

The data now look like those in Table 10.4 (WBEXP10_24).

Table 10.4   Excel dataset for drugs and procedures effect on percent stenosis. The nominal independent variables are represented with 0/1 indicator variables.

STENOIS	BYPASS	ANGIO
30	0	1
35	0	1
35	0	1
44	0	1
48	0	1
48	0	1
50	0	1
55	0	1
60	0	1
62	0	1
15	1	0
17	1	0
18	1	0
22	1	0
28	1	0
29	1	0
32	1	0
36	1	0
40	1	0
44	1	0
24	0	0
30	0	0
30	0	0
33	0	0
38	0	0
38	0	0
42	0	0
45	0	0
54	0	0
55	0	0

10.24. Analyze those data and interpret them

The following output is what we receive from the "Regression" Analysis Tool when we include serum cholesterol (CHOL) as a continuous independent variable, and indicator variables for the treatment groups. ANGIO is an indicator variable that is equal to one if the person had angioplasty and equal to zero otherwise. BYPASS is an indicator variable that is equal to one if the person had bypass surgery and equal to zero otherwise.

SUMMARY OUTPUT

Regression Statistics	
Multiple R	0.959976455
R Square	0.921554794
Adjusted R Square	0.912503424
Standard Error	3.748311358
Observations	30

ANOVA

	df	SS	MS	F	SignificanceF
Regression	3	4291.404211	1430.46807	101.8138477	1.71625E-14
Residual	26	365.295789	14.04983804		
Total	29	4656.7			

	Coefficients	Standard Error	t Stat	P-value	Lower 95%	Upper 95%
Intercept	0.265821992	3.104800618	0.085616445	0.932427231	-6.11618708	6.647831064
BYPASS	-14.21411443	1.695368915	-8.384083432	7.26071E-09	-17.69899514	-10.72923372
ANGIO	7.785220284	1.676296159	4.644298826	8.59577E-05	4.339544181	11.23089639
CHOLES	0.147797161	0.010977944	13.46309987	3.14249E-13	0.125231674	0.170362649

Since the indicator variables for BYPASS and ANGIO are significantly different from zero, the intercepts for BYPASS and ANGIO are significantly different from the intercept for stent. Since the regression coefficient for cholesterol is positive and significant, percent stenosis increases as serum cholesterol increases.

10.25. Represent those relationships graphically

Those three regression lines have the same slope (i.e., they are parallel). To allow the lines to have different slopes, we need to add interactions between each of the indicator variables and the continuous independent variable to the regression equation. With interactions, the data are as in Table 10.5 (WBEXP10_26).

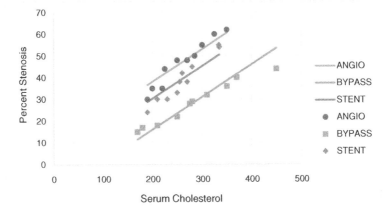

Figure 10.1. Scatter plot of the results in Example 10.24.

Table 10.5   Excel dataset for drugs, procedures, and serum cholesterol effect on percent stenosis. The nominal independent variables are represented with 0/1 indicator variables and interactions.

DRUG	STENOIS	BYPASS	ANGIO	CHOLES	BY*CHOL	AN*CHOL
DRUG1	30	0	1	190	0	190
DRUG1	35	0	1	200	0	200
DRUG1	35	0	1	220	0	220
DRUG2	44	0	1	225	0	225
DRUG1	48	0	1	250	0	250
DRUG2	48	0	1	270	0	270
DRUG2	50	0	1	285	0	285
DRUG2	55	0	1	300	0	300
DRUG1	60	0	1	325	0	325
DRUG2	62	0	1	350	0	350
DRUG2	15	1	0	170	170	0
DRUG2	17	1	0	180	180	0
DRUG1	18	1	0	210	210	0
DRUG2	22	1	0	250	250	0
DRUG2	28	1	0	275	275	0
DRUG1	29	1	0	280	280	0
DRUG2	32	1	0	310	310	0
DRUG1	36	1	0	350	350	0
DRUG1	40	1	0	370	370	0
DRUG1	44	1	0	450	450	0
DRUG1	24	0	0	190	0	0
DRUG1	30	0	0	210	0	0
DRUG1	30	0	0	230	0	0
DRUG1	33	0	0	250	0	0
DRUG2	38	0	0	255	0	0
DRUG2	38	0	0	270	0	0
DRUG2	42	0	0	260	0	0
DRUG1	45	0	0	280	0	0
DRUG2	54	0	0	335	0	0
DRUG2	55	0	0	334	0	0

10.26. Analyze and interpret those data

The slope of CHOL for BYPASS is lower than the slope of CHOL for STENT, The slope for ANGIO is higher than the slope for STENT.

10.27. Represent those data graphically

Since an interaction is created by multiplying two (or more) independent variables together, the interaction is highly correlated with those variables. Thus, there is the potential for collinearity. One effect of this is that it is harder to interpret the regression coefficients for the independent variables that are part of the interaction as long as the interaction is in the regression equation. For this reason, interactions can be dropped from the regression equation if they are not statistically significant.

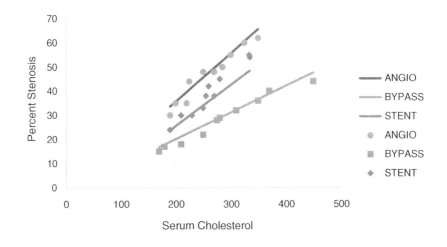

Figure 10.2. Scatter plot of the results in Example 10.26.

10.28. Analyze and interpret the data with the interaction between ANGI and cholesterol removed. What happens? Why?

The P-values got smaller because some collinearity was removed.

EXERCISES

10.1. Suppose we are interested in the relationship between dietary sodium intake (NA) and diastolic blood pressure (DBP). To investigate this relationship, we measure both for a sample of 40 persons. Because DBP and NA both increase with age, we decide to control for age in our analysis. The data for this question are in the Excel file: EXR10_1. Based on those observations, which of the following is closest to the percent variation in DBP that is explained by the combination of NA and age?

    A. 14.4%

    B. 24.3%

    C. 30.7%

    D. 38.0%

    E. 55.4%

10.2. Suppose we are interested in which blood chemistry measurements are predictive of urine creatinine. To investigate this, we identify 100 persons and measure their urine creatinine levels. We also measure serum creatinine, blood urea nitrogen (BUN), and serum potassium. These data are in the Excel file called EXR10_2. Use Excel to determine the percent of the variation in urine creatinine that is explained by the combination of serum creatinine, BUN, and serum potassium. Which of the following is closest to that value?

A. 73.3%

B. 69.3%

C. 53.7%

D. 48.0%

E. 43.0%

10.3. Suppose we are interested in the relationship between dietary sodium intake (NA) and diastolic blood pressure (DBP). To investigate this relationship, we measure both for a sample of 40 persons. Because DBP and NA both increase with age, we decide to control for age in our analysis. The data for this question is in the Excel file: EXR10_1. Based on those observations, test the null hypothesis that the combination of NA and age does not help estimate DBP, versus the alternative hypothesis that it does. If you allow a 5% chance of making a type I error, which of the following is the best conclusion to draw?

A. Reject both the null and alternative hypotheses

B. Accept both the null and alternative hypotheses

C. Reject the null hypothesis and accept the alternative hypothesis

D. Accept the null hypothesis and reject the alternative hypothesis

E. It is best not to draw a conclusion about the null and alternative hypotheses from these observations

10.4. Suppose we are interested in which blood chemistry measurements are predictive of urine creatinine. To investigate this, we identify 100 persons and measure their urine creatinine levels. We also measure serum creatinine, blood urea nitrogen (BUN), and serum potassium. These data are in the Excel file called EXR10_2. Use Excel to test the null hypothesis that the combination of serum creatinine, BUN, and serum potassium do not help estimate urine creatinine versus the alternative hypothesis that they do help. If you allow a 5% chance of making a type I error, what is the best conclusion to draw?

A. Reject both the null and alternative hypotheses

B. Accept both the null and alternative hypotheses

C. Reject the null hypothesis and accept the alternative hypothesis

D. Accept the null hypothesis and reject the alternative hypothesis

E. It is best not to draw a conclusion about the null and alternative hypotheses from these observations

10.5. Suppose we are interested in the relationship between dietary sodium intake (NA) and diastolic blood pressure (DBP). To investigate this relationship, we measure both for a sample of 40 persons. Because DBP and NA both increase with age, we decide to control for age in our analysis. The data for this question is in the Excel file: EXR10_1. Based on those observations, test the null hypothesis that the regression coefficient for NA, controlling for AGE, is equal to zero in the population versus the alternative hypothesis that it is not equal to zero. If you allow a 5% chance of making a type I error, which of the following is the best conclusion to draw?

A. Reject both the null and alternative hypotheses

B. Accept both the null and alternative hypotheses

C. Reject the null hypothesis and accept the alternative hypothesis

D. Accept the null hypothesis and reject the alternative hypothesis

E. It is best not to draw a conclusion about the null and alternative hypotheses from these observations

10.6. Suppose we are interested in which blood chemistry measurements are predictive of urine creatinine. To investigate this, we identify 100 persons and measure their urine creatinine levels. We also measure serum creatinine, blood urea nitrogen (BUN), and serum potassium. These data are in the Excel file called EXR10_2. Use Excel to test the null hypothesis that the regression coefficient for serum creatinine, when controlling for BUN and serum potassium, is equal to zero versus the alternative hypothesis that it is not equal to zero. If you allow a 5% chance of making a type I error, what is the best conclusion to draw?

A. Reject both the null and alternative hypotheses

B. Accept both the null and alternative hypotheses

C. Reject the null hypothesis and accept the alternative hypothesis

D. Accept the null hypothesis and reject the alternative hypothesis

E. It is best not to draw a conclusion about the null and alternative hypotheses from these observations

10.7. Suppose we are interested in the relationship between dietary sodium intake (NA) and diastolic blood pressure (DBP). To investigate this relationship, we measure both for a sample of 40 persons. Because DBP and NA both increase with age, we decide to control for age in our analysis. The data for this question are in the Excel file: EXR10_1. Based on those observations, which of the following independent variables contributes the most to the estimate of DBP, controlling for the other independent variables?

A. AGE

B. NA

C. They both contribute about the same to estimation of DBP

10.8. Suppose we are interested in which blood chemistry measurements are predictive of urine creatinine. To investigate this, we identify 100 persons and measure their urine creatinine levels. We also measure serum creatinine, blood urea nitrogen (BUN), and serum potassium. These data are in the Excel file called EXR10_2. Use Excel to determine which of the independent variables contributes the most to estimation of urine creatinine, while controlling for the other independent variables?

A. Serum creatinine

B. BUN

C. Serum potassium

D. They all contribute about the same to estimation of urine creatinine

10.9. Suppose we are interested in the survival time for persons with cancer of various organs. To investigate this, we identify 64 persons who died with cancer as the primary cause of death and record the period of time from their initial diagnosis to their death (in days). Those data are in the Excel file EXR10_3. Based on those data, test the null hypothesis that all five means are equal to the same value in the population versus the alternative that they are not all equal. If you allow a 5% chance of making a type I error, which of the following is the best conclusion to draw?

A. Reject both the null and alternative hypotheses

B. Accept both the null and alternative hypotheses

C. Reject the null hypothesis and accept the alternative hypothesis

D. Accept the null hypothesis and reject the alternative hypothesis

E. It is best not to draw a conclusion about the null and alternative hypotheses from these observations

10.10. Suppose we are interested in force of head impact for crash dummies in vehicles with different driver safety equipment. To study this relationship, we examine the results for 175 tests. Those data are in the Excel file: EXR10_4. Based on those data, test the null hypothesis that all four means are equal to the same value in the population versus the alternative that they are not all equal. If you allow a 5% chance of making a type I error, which of the following is the best conclusion to draw?

A. Reject both the null and alternative hypotheses

B. Accept both the null and alternative hypotheses

C. Reject the null hypothesis and accept the alternative hypothesis

D. Accept the null hypothesis and reject the alternative hypothesis

E. It is best not to draw a conclusion about the null and alternative hypotheses from these observations

10.11. Suppose we are interested in survival times for persons with cancer of various organs. To investigate this, we identify 64 persons who died with cancer as the primary cause of death and record the period of time from their initial diagnosis to their death (in days). Those data are in the Excel file: EXR10_3. Based on those data, perform tests comparing two means at a time in a way that avoids problems with multiple comparisons. If you allow a 5% chance of making a type I error, which of the following is the best conclusion to draw?

A. All five means are significantly different from each other

B. The mean for Bronchus is significantly different from all of the other means

C. The mean for Bronchus is significantly different from all of the other means except the mean for Stomach

D. The mean for Breast is significantly different from all of the other means

E. The mean for Breast is significantly different from all of the other means except the mean for Ovary

10.12. Suppose we are interested in force of head impact for crash dummies in vehicles with different driver safety equipment. To study this relationship, we examine the results for 175 tests. Those data are in the Excel file: EXR10_4. Based on those data, perform tests comparing two means at a time in a way that avoids problems with multiple comparisons. If you allow a 5% chance of making a type I error, which of the following is the best conclusion to draw?

A. All four means are significantly different from each other

B. Manual Belt is significantly different from the other three means, but the other three means are not significantly different from each other

C. All four means are significantly different from each other except Airbag and Motorized belt

D. All four means are significantly different from each other except Motorized Belt and Passive Belt

E. All four means are significantly different from each other except Passive Belt and Manual Belt

10.13. In a study of clinical depression, patients were randomly assigned to one of four drug groups (three active drugs and a placebo) and to a cognitive therapy group (active versus placebo). The dependent variable is a difference between scores on a depression questionnaire. The results are in the Excel file: EXR10_5. Based on those data, test the null hypothesis of no interaction between drug and therapy versus the alternative hypothesis that there is interaction allowing a 5% chance of making a type I error. Which of the following is the best conclusion to draw?

A. Reject both the null and alternative hypotheses

B. Accept both the null and alternative hypotheses

C. Reject the null hypothesis and accept the alternative hypothesis

D. Accept the null hypothesis and reject the alternative hypothesis

    E. It is best not to draw a conclusion about the null and alternative hypotheses from these observations

10.14. In a multicenter study of a new treatment for hypertension, patients at nine centers were randomly assigned to a new treatment or standard treatment. The dependent variable is a difference in diastolic blood pressure from a pretreatment value. The results are in the Excel file: EXR10_6. Based on those data, test the null hypothesis of no interaction between drug and center versus the alternative hypothesis that there is interaction allowing a 5% chance of making a type I error. Which of the following is the best conclusion to draw?

    A. Reject both the null and alternative hypotheses

    B. Accept both the null and alternative hypotheses

    C. Reject the null hypothesis and accept the alternative hypothesis

    D. Accept the null hypothesis and reject the alternative hypothesis

    E. It is best not to draw a conclusion about the null and alternative hypotheses from these observations

10.15. In a study of clinical depression, patients were randomly assigned to one of four drug groups (three active drugs and a placebo) and to a cognitive therapy group (active versus no therapy). The dependent variable is a difference between scores on a depression questionnaire. The results are in the Excel file: EXR10_5. Based on those data, test the null hypothesis of no differences between drug groups versus the alternative hypothesis that there is a difference, ignoring the possibility of an interaction. Allowing a 5% chance of making a type I error, which of the following is the best conclusion to draw?

    A. Reject both the null and alternative hypotheses

    B. Accept both the null and alternative hypotheses

    C. Reject the null hypothesis and accept the alternative hypothesis

    D. Accept the null hypothesis and reject the alternative hypothesis

    E. It is best not to draw a conclusion about the null and alternative hypotheses from these observations

10.16. In a multicenter study of a new treatment for hypertension, patients at nine centers were randomly assigned to a new treatment or standard treatment. The dependent variable is a difference in diastolic blood pressure from a pretreatment value. The results are in the Excel file: EXR10_6. Based on those data, test the null hypothesis of no difference between drugs versus the alternative hypothesis that there is a difference, ignoring the possibility of an interaction. If you allow a 5% chance of making a type I error, which of the following is the best conclusion to draw?

    A. Reject both the null and alternative hypotheses

    B. Accept both the null and alternative hypotheses

C. Reject the null hypothesis and accept the alternative hypothesis

D. Accept the null hypothesis and reject the alternative hypothesis

E. It is best not to draw a conclusion about the null and alternative hypotheses from these observations

10.17. In a study of clinical depression, patients were randomly assigned to one of four drug groups (three active drugs and a placebo) and to a cognitive therapy group (active versus no therapy). The dependent variable is a difference between scores on a depression questionnaire. The results are in the Excel file: EXR10_5. Based on those data, test the null hypothesis of no difference between therapy groups versus the alternative hypothesis that there is a difference, ignoring the possibility of an interaction. Allowing a 5% chance of making a type I error, which of the following is the best conclusion to draw?

A. Reject both the null and alternative hypotheses

B. Accept both the null and alternative hypotheses

C. Reject the null hypothesis and accept the alternative hypothesis

D. Accept the null hypothesis and reject the alternative hypothesis

E. It is best not to draw a conclusion about the null and alternative hypotheses from these observations

10.18. In a multicenter study of a new treatment for hypertension, patients at nine centers were randomly assigned to a new treatment or standard treatment. The dependent variable is a difference in diastolic blood pressure from a pretreatment value. The results are in the Excel file: EXR10_6. Based on those data, test the null hypothesis of no difference among centers in the population versus the alternative hypothesis that there is a difference, ignoring the possibility of an interaction. If you allow a 5% chance of making a type I error, which of the following is the best conclusion to draw?

A. Reject both the null and alternative hypotheses

B. Accept both the null and alternative hypotheses

C. Reject the null hypothesis and accept the alternative hypothesis

D. Accept the null hypothesis and reject the alternative hypothesis

E. It is best not to draw a conclusion about the null and alternative hypotheses from these observations

10.19. Suppose we are interested in the relationship between body mass index (BMI) and serum cholesterol (the dependent variable) controlling for gender ($SEX = 1$ for women and $SEX = 0$ for men). To study this relationship, we analyze data from 300 persons who participated in the Framingham Heart Study. Those data are in Excel file: EXR10_7. Analyze those data as an ANCOVA. From that output, do you think the slopes of the regression lines for men and women are different?

A. No, the slopes are the same

B. Yes, the slopes are different, but not significantly different

C. Yes, the slopes are different and they are significantly different

10.20. Suppose we are interested in the relationship between time since diagnosis of HIV and CD4 count. To investigate this relationship, we examine 1,151 HIV positive patients. In making this comparison, we control for gender (SEX = 1 for women and SEX = 0 for men). These data are in the Excel file: EXR10_8. Which of the following is the best description of the relationship between time since diagnosis and CD4 in the sample?

A. CD4 decreases with longer time since diagnosis for both men and women

B. CD4 decreases with longer time since diagnosis for women only

C. CD4 decreases with longer time since diagnosis for men only

D. CD4 decreases with longer time since diagnosis for men and increases for women

E. CD4 decreases with longer time since diagnosis for women and increases for men

CHAPTER 11

Multivariable Analysis of an Ordinal Dependent Variable

CHAPTER SUMMARY

When we have an ordinal dependent variable, we can examine that variable relative to more than one nominal independent variables. Statistical procedures for an ordinal dependent variable and more than one nominal independent variable are very similar in operation and interpretation to procedures for continuous dependent variables. A parallel procedure to a one-way analysis of variance is the Kruskal-Wallis test. The test statistic for the Kruskal-Wallis test (H) is calculated from the between sum of squares and total mean square when ANOVA procedures are performed on ranks.

Kruskal-Wallis test statistics calculated from a sample's observations can be compared to values in Table B.9 to test the omnibus null hypothesis. This is parallel to the F-ratio test in analysis of variance. If the numbers of observations in

Workbook to Accompany Introduction to Biostatistical Applications in Health Research with Microsoft® Office Excel®, First Edition. Robert P. Hirsch.
© 2016 John Wiley & Sons, Inc. Published 2016 by John Wiley & Sons, Inc.

each group are greater than the values in Table B.9, the Kruskal-Wallis test statistic can be considered to be a chi-square value with degrees of freedom equal to the number of groups minus one and compared to values in Table B.7.

When the dependent variable is continuous, we usually use a procedure such as the Student-Newman-Keuls test to compare two groups of values of the dependent variable. When the dependent variable is ordinal, we use a parallel procedure that we call Dunn's test. Dunn's test is very much like the Student-Newman-Keuls test except that the means of the ranks of the dependent variable values are compared rather than the means of the values of the dependent variable values themselves. The test statistic in Dunn's procedure is compared to values in Table B.10 to test the null hypothesis that the difference is equal to zero in the population from which the sample was drawn.

To perform an analysis that is parallel to factorial analysis of variance for continuous dependent variables on ordinal dependent variables, we take advantage of the fact that the Kruskal-Wallis test statistic can be calculated by dividing the between sum of squares for the ranks of values of the dependent variable by the total mean square for those ranks.

When we have more than one factor among the independent variables, we can partition the between sum of squares for the ranks in the same way that we partitioned the between sum of squares in factorial analysis of variance. Null hypotheses that the means of the ranks of the categories within each factor are equal or that there is no interaction between factors in the population can be tested by dividing the appropriate partition of the between sum of squares by the total mean square and comparing the resulting test statistic to the values in Table B.9.

GLOSSARY

Dunn's Test – a nonparametric posterior test for comparison of two groups of ordinal dependent variable values at a time.

Kruskal-Wallis Test – a nonparametric method for one-way and factorial ANOVAs.

EQUATIONS

$H = \frac{\text{Between Sum of Squares}}{\text{Total Mean Square}}$
Kruskal-Wallis test statistic for one-way ANOVA. (see Equation {11.1})

$H = \frac{\text{Main Effect Sum of Squares}}{\text{Total Mean Square}}$
Kruskal-Wallis test statistic for a main effect in factorial ANOVA. See Equation {11.2})

$H = \frac{\text{Interaction Sum of Squares}}{\text{Total Mean Square}}$
Kruskal-Wallis test statistic for an interaction in factorial ANOVA. (see Equation{11.3})

$Q = \frac{\left(\bar{Y}_{\text{Rank}_1} \bar{Y}_{\text{Rank}_2}\right) - \left(\mu_{\text{Rank}_1} - \mu_{\text{Rank}_2}\right)}{\sqrt{\frac{\text{TMS}}{n_1} + \frac{\text{TMS}}{n_2}}}$
Dunn's test. (see Equation {11.4})

EXAMPLES

In Chapter 10, we were interested in comparing three treatments for coronary heart disease: (1) bypass surgery, (2) stent implantation, and (3) balloon angioplasty. To do this, we randomly assigned 30 persons to one of the three treatment groups (10 per group). Six months after treatment, we measured the percent stenosis of the treated artery. We observed the results in Table 11.1 (WBEXP10_17).

Table 11.1   Excel table of stenosis data.

	BYPASS	STENT	ANGIO
DRUG1	28	30	48
DRUG1	15	45	35
DRUG1	22	24	30
DRUG1	17	33	35
DRUG1	32	30	60
DRUG2	40	55	55
DRUG2	36	38	44
DRUG2	44	42	62
DRUG2	29	54	50
DRUG2	18	38	48

The null hypothesis we tested is that the means in the groups are all equal to the same value in the population. Now, let us analyze these data on an ordinal scale.

11.1. Rank those data values in preparation for the Kruskal-Wallis test

The data are ranked without regard to which group they belong.

Table 11.2   Excel table of ranked stenosis data.

	BYPASS	STENT	ANGIO
DRUG1	6	9	23.5
DRUG1	1	22	13.5
DRUG1	4	5	9
DRUG1	2	12	13.5
DRUG1	11	9	29
DRUG2	18	27.5	27.5
DRUG2	15	16.5	20.5
DRUG2	20.5	19	30
DRUG2	7	26	25
DRUG2	3	16.5	23.5

The easiest way to rank these data is to use the "rank.avg" function.

11.2. Test the null hypothesis that the mean of the ranks is the same for all three procedure groups

To test this null hypothesis, we use the "Anova: Single Factor" analysis tool.

Anova: Single Factor

SUMMARY

Groups	Count	Sum	Average	Variance
BYPASS	10	87.5	8.75	48.84722222
STENT	10	162.5	16.25	56.90277778
ANGIO	10	215	21.5	52.22222222

ANOVA

Source of Variation	SS	df	MS	F	P-value	F crit
Between Groups	821.25	2	410.625	7.79804818	0.002122846	3.354130829
Within Groups	1421.75	27	52.65740741			
Total	2243	29				

Then, we use the information from that output to calculate the Kruskal-Wallis test statistic. Using Equation {11.1}, we get:

$$H = \frac{\text{Between Sum of Squares}}{\text{Total Mean Square}} = \frac{821.25}{2,243/29} = 10.618$$

That value can be interpreted by comparing it to a chi-square with degrees of freedom equal to the between variation (i.e., two). That chi-square is equal to 5.991. Since the calculated value is greater than the critical value, we can reject the null hypothesis that all three groups have the same mean of the ranks in the population.

11.3. Use Dunn's test to determine which procedure groups are significantly different

To begin, we array the means of the ranks in numeric order:

Table 11.3   Stenosis means in ascending order.

BYPASS	STENT	ANGIO
8.75	16.25	21.50

The first comparison we make is between BYPASS and ANGIO. Using Equation {11.4}, we get:

$$Q = \frac{(\overline{Y}_{rank_1} - \overline{Y}_{rank_2}) - (\mu_{rank_1} - \mu_{rank_2})}{\sqrt{\frac{TMS}{n_1} + \frac{TMS}{n_2}}} = \frac{(8.75 - 21.50) - 0}{\sqrt{\frac{2,243/29}{10} + \frac{2,243/29}{10}}} = -3.24$$

We compare this to a critical value from Table B.10. For $k = 3$ and $\alpha = 0.05$, the critical value is 2.394. Since the absolute value of the calculated value (3.24) is greater than the critical value (2.394), we reject the null hypothesis that mean ranks for BYPASS and ANGIO are equal in the population. This also allows us to compare BYPASS to STENT and STENT to ANGIO.

For the comparison of BYPASS to STENT and STENT to ANGIO, we observe the following:

$$Q = \frac{(\overline{Y}_{rank_1} - \overline{Y}_{rank_2}) - (\mu_{rank_1} - \mu_{rank_2})}{\sqrt{\frac{TMS}{n_1} + \frac{TMS}{n_2}}} = \frac{(8.75 - 16.25) - 0}{\sqrt{\frac{2,243/29}{10} + \frac{2,243/29}{10}}} = -1.91$$

$$Q = \frac{(\overline{Y}_{rank_1} - \overline{Y}_{rank_2}) - (\mu_{rank_1} - \mu_{rank_2})}{\sqrt{\frac{TMS}{n_1} + \frac{TMS}{n_2}}} = \frac{(16.25 - 21.50) - 0}{\sqrt{\frac{2,243/29}{10} + \frac{2,243/29}{10}}} = -1.33$$

The critical value from Table B.10 for $k = 2$ and $\alpha = 0.05$ is 1.96. Since the absolute calculated values are less than this critical value, we fail to reject the null hypotheses that the mean ranks are equal in the population.

Now, we include two drug groups along with the three procedures for Examples 11.4-11.6. We need to analyze the ranks using the "Anova: Two-Factor With Replication" analysis tool.

Anova: Two-Factor With Replication

SUMMARY	BYPASS	STENT	ANGIO	Total
DRUG1				
Count	5	5	5	15
Sum	24	57	88.5	169.5
Average	4.8	11.4	17.7	11.3
Variance	15.7	41.3	68.075	65.45714286
DRUG2				
Count	5	5	5	15
Sum	63.5	105.5	126.5	295.5
Average	12.7	21.1	25.3	19.7
Variance	55.2	27.925	13.325	56.95714286
Total				
Count	10	10	10	
Sum	87.5	162.5	215	
Average	8.75	16.25	21.5	
Variance	48.84722222	56.90277778	52.22222222	

ANOVA						
Source of Variation	SS	df	MS	F	P-value	F crit
Sample	529.2	1	529.2	14.33337095	0.000903354	4.259677273
Columns	821.25	2	410.625	11.12176955	0.000381876	3.402826105
Interaction	6.45	2	3.225	0.087349058	0.916647138	3.402826105
Within	886.1	24	36.92083333			
Total	2243	29				

11.4. Test the null hypothesis that there is no interaction between procedure and drug

From that output, we calculate the Kruskal-Wallis test statistic for the interaction using Equation {11.3}:

$$H = \frac{\text{Interaction Sum of Squares}}{\text{Total Mean Square}} = \frac{6.45}{2,243/29} = 0.083$$

The critical value from Table B.7 is 5.991. Since the calculated value (0.083) is less than the critical value, we fail to reject the null hypothesis of no interaction. This indicates it makes sense to interpret the main effects.

11.5. Test the null hypothesis that the mean of the ranks is the same for all three procedure groups

This is the main effect of procedure. The procedures were separated into columns in the dataset, so the sum of squares for procedure are labeled "Columns" by Excel. Using Equation {11.2}:

$$H = \frac{\text{Columns Sum of Squares}}{\text{Total Mean Square}} = \frac{821.25}{2,243/29} = 10.618$$

The critical value from Table B.7 is 5.991. Since the calculated value (10.618) is greater than the critical value (5.991), we reject this null hypothesis.

11.6. Test the null hypothesis that the mean of the ranks is the same for both drug groups

This is the main effect of drug. The drugs were separated in rows of the dataset. Excel calls this the "Sample" variation. Using Equation {11.2}:

$$H = \frac{\text{Samples Sum of Squares}}{\text{Total Mean Square}} = \frac{529.2}{2,243/29} = 6.842$$

There is only one "Samples" degree of freedom, so the critical value from Table B.7 is 3.841. Since the calculated value (6.842) is greater than the critical value (3.841), we reject this null hypothesis.

EXERCISES

11.1. In a study of clinical depression, patients were randomly assigned to one of four drug groups (three active drugs and a placebo) and to cognitive therapy (versus no therapy). The dependent variable is a difference between scores on a depression questionnaire. The results are in the Excel file: EXR10_5. Based on those data, test the null hypothesis of no interaction between drug and therapy versus the alternative hypothesis that there is interaction without assuming a Gaussian sampling distribution. Allowing a 5% chance of making a type I error, which of the following is the best conclusion to draw?

A. Reject both the null and alternative hypotheses

B. Accept both the null and alternative hypotheses

C. Reject the null hypothesis and accept the alternative hypothesis

D. Accept the null hypothesis and reject the alternative hypothesis

E. It is best not to draw a conclusion about the null and alternative hypotheses from these observations

11.2. In a multicenter study of a new treatment for hypertension, patients at nine centers were randomly assigned to a new treatment or standard treatment. The dependent variable is a difference in diastolic blood pressure from a pretreatment value. The results are in the Excel file: EXR10_6. Based on those data, test the null hypothesis of no interaction between drug and center versus the alternative hypothesis that there is interaction without assuming a Gaussian sampling distribution. Allowing a 5% chance of making a type I error, which of the following is the best conclusion to draw?

A. Reject both the null and alternative hypotheses

B. Accept both the null and alternative hypotheses

C. Reject the null hypothesis and accept the alternative hypothesis

D. Accept the null hypothesis and reject the alternative hypothesis

E. It is best not to draw a conclusion about the null and alternative hypotheses from these observations

11.3. In a study of clinical depression, patients were randomly assigned to one of four drug groups (three active drugs and a placebo) and to cognitive therapy (versus no therapy). The dependent variable is a difference between scores on a depression questionnaire. The results are in the Excel file: EXR10_5. Based on those data, test the null hypothesis of no differences between drug groups versus the alternative hypothesis that there is a difference, ignoring the possibility of an interaction and not assuming a Gaussian sampling distribution. Allowing a 5% chance of making a type I error, which of the following is the best conclusion to draw?

A. Reject both the null and alternative hypotheses

B. Accept both the null and alternative hypotheses

C. Reject the null hypothesis and accept the alternative hypothesis

D. Accept the null hypothesis and reject the alternative hypothesis

    E. It is best not to draw a conclusion about the null and alternative hypotheses from these observations

11.4. In a multicenter study of a new treatment for hypertension, patients at nine centers were randomly assigned to a new treatment or standard treatment. The dependent variable is a difference in diastolic blood pressure from a pretreatment value. The results are in the Excel file: EXR10_6. Based on those data, test the null hypothesis of no difference between drugs versus the alternative hypothesis that there is a difference, ignoring the possibility of an interaction and not assuming a Gaussian sampling distribution. If you allow a 5% chance of making a type I error, which of the following is the best conclusion to draw?

    A. Reject both the null and alternative hypotheses

    B. Accept both the null and alternative hypotheses

    C. Reject the null hypothesis and accept the alternative hypothesis

    D. Accept the null hypothesis and reject the alternative hypothesis

    E. It is best not to draw a conclusion about the null and alternative hypotheses from these observations

11.5. In a study of clinical depression, patients were randomly assigned to one of four drug groups (three active drugs and a placebo) and to cognitive therapy (versus no therapy). The dependent variable is a difference between scores on a depression questionnaire. The results are in the Excel file: EXR10_5. Based on those data, test the null hypothesis of no differences between therapy groups versus the alternative hypothesis that there is a difference, ignoring the possibility of an interaction and not assuming a Gaussian sampling distribution. Allowing a 5% chance of making a type I error, which of the following is the best conclusion to draw?

    A. Reject both the null and alternative hypotheses

    B. Accept both the null and alternative hypotheses

    C. Reject the null hypothesis and accept the alternative hypothesis

    D. Accept the null hypothesis and reject the alternative hypothesis

    E. It is best not to draw a conclusion about the null and alternative hypotheses from these observations

11.6. In a multicenter study of a new treatment for hypertension, patients at nine centers were randomly assigned to a new treatment or standard treatment. The dependent variable is a difference in diastolic blood pressure from a pretreatment value. The results are in the Excel file: EXR10_6. Based on those data, test the null hypothesis of no difference among centers in the population versus the alternative hypothesis that there is a difference, ignoring the possibility of an interaction and not assuming a Gaussian sampling distribution. If you allow a 5% chance of making a type I error, which of the following is the best conclusion to draw?

A. Reject both the null and alternative hypotheses
B. Accept both the null and alternative hypotheses
C. Reject the null hypothesis and accept the alternative hypothesis
D. Accept the null hypothesis and reject the alternative hypothesis
E. It is best not to draw a conclusion about the null and alternative hypotheses from these observations

CHAPTER 12

Multivariable Analysis of a Nominal Dependent Variable

CHAPTER SUMMARY

We have two choices for our basic approach to multivariable analysis of a nominal dependent variable. One approach that is applicable to continuous and/or nominal independent variables is comparable to multiple regression analysis for a continuous dependent variable. The other approach is stratified analysis, which can be performed only with nominal independent variables or independent variables converted to a nominal scale.

In the regression approach to the analysis of nominal dependent variables, there are two techniques we encounter most often in health research. When the nominal dependent variable is expressed as a probability or as odds, we use logistic regression. Logistic regression uses a transformation of the nominal dependent variable known as the logit transformation. The logit transformation is equal to the

Workbook to Accompany Introduction to Biostatistical Applications in Health Research with Microsoft® Office Excel®, First Edition. Robert P. Hirsch.
© 2016 John Wiley & Sons, Inc. Published 2016 by John Wiley & Sons, Inc.

natural logarithm of the ratio of the probabilities of an event and its complement. This is the same as the natural logarithm of the odds of the dependent variable (known as the log odds).

To estimate values of the logit transformed dependent variable, logistic regression analysis uses a linear combination of the independent variables that is the same as in multiple regression analysis of continuous dependent variables.

There are two ways in which the estimated values of the dependent variable in logistic regression can be expressed. One way is by estimating probabilities for specific values of all the independent variables. The other way to interpret estimated values of the dependent variable in logistic regression is by estimating odds ratios for specific values of the independent variables, one at a time.

Cox regression is the regression approach that is most often used when the nominal dependent variable is affected by time and expressed as a rate. The dependent variable in the Cox regression equation is the natural logarithm of the rate.

It is possible to interpret the estimated values of the dependent variable in Cox regression as the rate corresponding to specific values for all the independent variables, but this is a little complicated since the "intercept" is a function of time. More often, dependent variable values are interpreted as a rate ratio corresponding to the regression coefficient for a specific independent variable.

Both logistic regression and Cox regression rely on the maximum likelihood method for estimating values of regression coefficients and testing hypotheses. In the maximum likelihood method, values for the coefficients are chosen so that the probability of obtaining the sample's observations from a population with those coefficients is as high as possible. Hypothesis testing in logistic and Cox regression uses a likelihood ratio. That likelihood ratio contains the probability of obtaining the sample's observations if the null hypothesis were true in the numerator and the probability of obtaining those observations if the population' coefficients were equal to the sample's estimates of those coefficients in the denominator.

The likelihood ratio can be used to test the omnibus null hypothesis that all the coefficients are equal to zero, or a partial likelihood ratio can be used to test the null hypothesis that a particular coefficient is equal to zero. These likelihood ratios differ in the likelihood used in their numerators. The likelihood ratio for the omnibus null hypothesis has in its numerator the likelihood of obtaining the observed data if all the coefficients were equal to zero. The partial likelihood ratio usually has in its numerator the likelihood of obtaining the observed data if a particular coefficient were equal to zero and all the other coefficients were equal to the values estimated from the sample's observations.

Regardless of which null hypothesis is being tested, evaluation of whether or not the likelihood ratio is unusual enough to allow rejection of the null hypothesis involves conversion of the likelihood ratio to a chi-square statistic. That chi-square value has degrees of freedom equal to the difference between the number of coefficients considered in the null hypothesis and the total number of coefficients in the regression equation.

When all the independent variables are nominal, we can still use logistic or Cox regression techniques to analyze them. An alternative to the regression approach for nominal independent variables, however, is the stratified analysis approach. In stratified analysis, we differentiate between one nominal independent variable that is of main interest and other independent variables that represent potential confounders. We then create a series of 2×2 tables, one for each value of the independent variable(s) representing the confounder(s).

With data that have been stratified, we have a choice of examining the relationship between the dependent variable and the independent variable of main interest within each of the strata separately or over all the strata combined. The choice between these two approaches depends on whether the relationship appears to be consistent over all the strata. When the relationship does not appear to be consistent over the strata, we choose to examine that relationship within each of the strata separately, using the techniques for bivariable analysis of a nominal dependent variable described in Chapter 9. If the relationship between the dependent variable and the main independent variable appears to be the same for all the strata (according to a test of homogeneity), we can facilitate interpretation of the relationship between the dependent variable and the independent variable of main interest by making one summary estimate by combining the estimates for each of the strata.

When it is more likely we will observe the nominal dependent variable event the longer we follow individuals and individuals in a study are followed for variable periods of time, we say the dependent variable is affected by time. In previous chapters, we have examined nominal dependent variables that are affected by time by estimating rates rather than probabilities. In this chapter, we examine an alternative approach to nominal dependent variables that are affected by time with a method called life-table analysis. In life-table analysis, follow-up time is treated like a nominal confounding variable used to create strata. Within each time stratum, the probability of surviving (i.e., avoiding the event) over the time interval is calculated. Of more interest than the probability of surviving (i.e., avoiding the event) a particular time stratum is the cumulative probability of surviving up to and including that time interval.

It is often of interest to compare the survival experience of two groups. Most commonly, entire life tables are compared graphically by examining survival plots. A survival plot graphs time on the abscissa (X-axis) and the cumulative probability of survival (i.e., avoiding the event) on the ordinate (Y-axis).

For both probabilities and rates, methods of interval estimation differ between differences and ratios. That is not true of hypothesis testing. The method we use to test the null hypothesis that the probability difference is equal to zero or that the probability or odds ratios are equal to one is an extension of the Mantel-Haenszel procedure first described in Chapter 9.

The Mantel-Haenszel procedure is also used to test the null hypothesis that two life tables are the same in the population from which the sample was drawn. Although the calculations are the same when a Mantel-Haenszel chi-square is calculated from data stratified by interval of follow-up, there is a feature of hypothesis testing in life-table analysis that is important to keep in mind. That feature is the number of observations in each time stratum becomes smaller as we consider strata for longer time intervals.

GLOSSARY

Actuarial Method – in life table analysis, an assumption that persons withdraw from a study at a uniform rate and thus, contribute half of the information contributed by persons who do not withdraw. Also known as the Cutler-Ederer method.

Cox Regression Analysis – a regression analysis used to estimate rate ratios.

Cumulative Probability – in life table analysis, the probability of surviving (i.e., not having the event) up to and through a particular time period. An intersection calculated using the multiplication rule of probability theory.

Generalized Linear Model – a recognition that all analyses for a nominal dependent variable can be expressed as a regression equation with very similar results to other analyses.

Indicator Variable – a numeric variable that has only qualitative value. Indicator variables are used to represent nominal variables in regression analyses.

Interaction Variable – a variable created by multiplying an indicator variable by another variable. It allows a different relationship between the other variable and dependent variable for different values of the indicator variable.

Kaplan-Meier Method – a method of life table analysis in which persons who withdraw in a particular time period are assumed to withdraw at the end of the period.

Least Squares Estimation – a method of deriving estimates that aims to minimize the squared differences between observed and estimated values of the dependent variable.

Life Table Analysis – a type of analysis that estimates risks from nominal dependent variables that are affected by time. It accomplishes this by stratifying the data by time.

Likelihood – the probability of obtaining the observations in the sample given the population's parameter(s) are equal to the sample's estimate(s). A type of conditional probability.

Likelihood Ratio – a ratio of two likelihoods (conditional probabilities) that represent different collections of independent variables.

Maximum Likelihood Estimation – a method of determining estimates that aims to maximize the likelihood of obtaining the sample's observations assuming the population's parameters are equal to the sample's estimates.

Logistic Regression – a regression analysis designed for nominal dependent variables not affected by time. It is characterized by the dependent variable being transformed using the logit transformation.

Logit Transformation – a mathematic representation of a probability in which the probability is changed to odds and then the natural logarithm is taken of the odds.

Log-Rank Test – the Mantel-Haenszel test applied to a nominal dependent variable stratified by time.

Mantel-Haenszel Estimate – a summary estimate in stratified analysis developed algebraically from strata-specific observations.

Mantel-Haenszel Test – a chi-square test that can be used to combine information among strata to test a null hypothesis about a summary estimate.

Precision-Based Estimate – a summary estimate in stratified analysis developed by taking a weighted average of strata-specific estimates using precision of the estimate as the weights.

Residual Confounding – incomplete control of a confounder, most often seen when controlling for a continuous confounder.

Sigmoid Curve – an S-shaped relationship between a probability and one (or more) continuous independent variables. A sigmoid curve approaches, but never crosses, zero and one. It is created by using a transformation, such as the logit transformation.

Strata – groups of dependent variable values in which all persons have the same value of the confounder(s).

Stratified Analysis – a method of controlling confounding by dividing the data into groups (strata) within which all persons have the same value of the confounder(s).

Strata-Specific Estimate – an estimate made using only the data in one stratum in stratified analysis.

Study-Relative Time – time determined from the point at which a person enters the study. It tells us how long a person has been in the study, regardless of the date on which (s)he entered the study.

Summary Estimate – in stratified analysis, a single estimate that represents the relationship between the dependent and independent variables regardless of strata.

Survival Plot ("Curve") – a graphic method of life table analysis that tracks the number of persons without the event over time.

Test of Homogeneity – in stratified analysis, a test of the null hypothesis that there is no difference among strata-specific values in the population. Failure to reject this null hypothesis means it makes sense to interpret a summary estimate, instead of strata-specific estimates.

Transformation – changing the dependent variable (or estimate) to a different mathematic form to facilitate analysis.

EQUATIONS

$p(\text{sample's data}|\beta = b)$

a likelihood. (see Equation {12.1})

$$LR = \frac{p(\text{sample's data}|\beta = b) \text{ for reduced model}}{p(\text{sample's data}|\beta = b) \text{ for full model}}$$

likelihood ratio. {see Equation {12.3})

$$\ln \frac{\theta}{1 - \theta} = \alpha + (\beta_1 \cdot X_1) + (\beta_2 \cdot X_2) \\ + \cdots + (\beta_k \cdot X_k)$$

logistic regression equation in the population. (see Equation {12.4})

$$\theta \triangleq p = \frac{1}{1 + e^{-[a + b_1 \cdot X_1 + b_2 \cdot X_2 + \cdots + b_k \cdot X_k]}}$$

estimation of the probability from logistic regression. (see Equation {12.5})

$$OR = \frac{e^{\alpha + \beta_1 \cdot (X_1 + 1) + \beta_2 \cdot X_2 + \cdots + \beta_k X_k}}{e^{\alpha + \beta_1 \cdot X_1 + \beta_2 \cdot X_2 + \cdots + \beta_k X_k}} = e^{\beta_1} \triangleq \hat{OR} = e^{b_1}$$

estimation of the odds ratio for a specific value of X_1 from logistic regression analysis. (see Equation {12.7})

$$OR_\Delta = \frac{e^{\alpha + \beta_1 \cdot (X_1 + \Delta) + \beta_2 \cdot X_2 + \cdots + \beta_k X_k}}{e^{\alpha + \beta_1 \cdot X_1 + \beta_2 \cdot X_2 + \cdots + \beta_k X_k}} = e^{\beta_1 \cdot \Delta} \triangleq e^{b_1 \cdot \Delta}$$

estimation of the odds ratio for a range of values for X_1 from logistic regression analysis. (see Equation {12.8})

$$OR = \frac{e^{\alpha + \beta_1 \cdot (+1) + \beta_2 \cdot X_2 + \cdots + \beta_k X_k}}{e^{\alpha + \beta_1 \cdot (-1) + \beta_2 \cdot X_2 + \cdots + \beta_k X_k}} = \frac{e^{\beta_1 \cdot (+1)}}{e^{\beta_1 \cdot (-1)}} = e^{\beta_1 \cdot 2}$$

estimation of the odds ratio for a value of X_1 which is a $+1/-1$ indicator variable. (see Equation {12.9})

$$OR_\Delta = e^{(\beta_1 \cdot \Delta) + (\beta_3 \cdot \Delta \cdot X_2)} \triangleq \hat{OR}_\Delta = e^{(b_1 \cdot \Delta) + (b_3 \cdot \Delta \cdot X_2)}$$

estimation of the odds ratio for a value of X_1 which is in an interaction with X_2. (see Equation {12.10})

$$\ln(\text{rate}) = \alpha_t + \beta_1 X_1 + \beta_2 X_2 + \cdots + \beta_k X_k$$

Cox regression equation in the population. (see Equation {12.11})

$$OR \triangleq \overline{OR} = \frac{\sum\limits_{i=1}^{k} a_i \cdot d_i / n_i}{\sum\limits_{i=1}^{k} b_i \cdot c_i / n_i}$$

Mantel-Haenszel summary estimate of the odds ratio. (see Equation {12.13})

$$RR \triangleq \overline{RR} = \frac{\sum\limits_{i=1}^{k} a_i \cdot (c_i + d_i) / n_i}{\sum\limits_{i=1}^{k} c_i \cdot (a_i + b_i) / n_i}$$

Mantel-Haenszel summary estimate of the risk ratio. (see Equation {12.14})

$$\chi^2 = \sum_{i=1}^{k} \frac{(Y_i - Y)^2}{\frac{1}{w_i}}$$

chi-square test of homogeneity. (see Equation {12.15})

$$\chi^2_{1df} = \frac{\left(\sum_{i=1}^{k} a_i - \sum_{i=1}^{k} E(a_i)\right)^2}{\sum_{i=1}^{k} \frac{(a_i + b_i) \cdot (c_i + d_i) \cdot (a_i + c_i) \cdot (b_i + d_i)}{n_i^2 \cdot (n_i - 1)}}$$

Mantel-Haenszel chi-square test. (see Equation {12.16})

$$p(\overline{event}_{t_i} | \overline{event}_{t_{<i}}) = 1 - \frac{a_{t_i}}{n_{t_i}}$$

probability of avoiding the event during i^{th} time period using the Kaplan-Meier method (see Equation {12.17})

$$p(\overline{event}_{t_i} \text{ and } \overline{event}_{t_{<i}}) = \prod_{t=1}^{i} p(\overline{event}_{t_k} | \overline{event}_t)$$

cumulative probability of avoiding the event over t time periods. (see Equation {12.18})

$$\text{Risk}_i = 1 - p(\overline{event}_{t=i} \text{ and } \overline{event}_{t=i-1} \text{ and } \cdots \text{ and } \overline{event}_{t=1})$$

calculation of risk from life table information. (see Equation {12.19})

$$p(\overline{event}_{t=i} | \overline{event}_{t<i}) = 1 - \frac{a_{t=i}}{n_{t=i} - \frac{w_{t=i}}{2}}$$

probability of avoiding the event during i^{th} time period using the actuarial method. (see Equation {12.20})

EXAMPLES

12.1. What does the null hypothesis that the regression coefficient is equal to zero imply about the odds ratio in logistic regression?

The null hypothesis that the regression coefficient is equal to zero is the same as the null hypothesis that the odds ratio is equal to one.

Suppose we are interested in risk factors for coronary artery disease (CAD). We design a study in which 200 high-risk persons are examined and 55 are found to have CAD. The following table compares risk factors between those 55 persons with CAD and the 160 persons without CAD:

Table 12.1   Risk factors for coronary artery disease.

RISK FACTOR	CAD ($n = 55$)	No CAD ($n = 145$)
Smoking	24 (44%)	26 (18%)
Diabetes	16 (29%)	39 (27%)
Dietary Fat	158 ± 11.1[1]	119 ± 6.0
Dietary Sodium	144 ± 9.8	124 ± 5.7

[1]Mean $\pm$ SE

The dataset contains two indicator variables. SMOKE is equal to one for smokers and equal to zero for nonsmokers. DIABETES is equal to one if the person has been diagnosed with diabetes and equal to zero otherwise. These data are in the WBEXP12_1 dataset.

12.2. Analyze those data using the BMR "Logistic Regression" program. What output do we get?

Logistic Regression

Omnibus H0	Log Lkhd	Chi Sq	DF	P-value
Intercept Only	−128.092			
	−107.245	20.778	6	0.002011

Variable	Estimate	Chi Sq	DF	P-Value
Intercept	1.3643	13.995	1	0.000183
FAT	−0.0049	4.69	1	0.030339
NA	−0.0038	2.547	1	0.110504
SMOKE	1.007	7.269	1	0.007015
DIABETES	0.1176	0.098	1	0.754243

12.3. Use that output to test the null hypothesis that the combination of risk factors does not help estimate the odds of getting CAD.

This is the omnibus null hypothesis. To answer this question, we look at the first table in the output. The P-value for this test is 0.00020. Since this P-value is less than 0.05, we reject the omnibus hypothesis.

12.4. Use the output in Example 12.2 to determine the association between CAD and each of the risk factors while controlling for the effect of the other risk factors.

To answer this question, we look at the second table in the output. In that table we see that the odds of having CAD is significantly associated with smoking (P = 0.0070) and the level of fat in the diet (P = 0.0303). The associations of CAD with having diabetes (P = 0.7537) and the level of sodium in the diet (P = 0.1105) are not statistically significant.

12.5. Calculate odds ratios for a 25-unit change in dietary fat and a 25-unit change in dietary sodium.

For dietary fat, the regression coefficient is equal to −0.0049. So, the odds ratio for a 25-unit change in dietary fat is:

$$\text{Odds Ratio} = e^{b_1 \cdot \Delta} = e^{-0.0049 \cdot 25} = 0.8847$$

For dietary sodium, the regression coefficient is equal to -0.0038. So, the odds ratio for a 25-unit change in dietary sodium is:

$$\text{Odds Ratio} = e^{b_1 \cdot \Delta} = e^{-0.0038 \cdot 25} = 0.9091$$

In these logistic regression analysis exercises, we were interested in risk factors for coronary artery disease (CAD). Using those same data, let us suppose we focus our interest on the relationship between diabetes and CAD. If we were to analyze the data with only these two nominal variables, we could summarize the data in a single 2×2 table:

		CAD		
		YES	NO	
Diabetes	YES	16	39	55
	NO	39	106	145

This is a bivariable analysis. We learned in Chapter 9 that we can summarize data like these using a probability difference, a probability ratio, or an odds ratio.

12.6. Determine the probability difference, probability ratio, and odds ratio for those data.

Using the BAHR "2 x 2 Table Analyzer" program:

Observed		Outcome		
		Yes	No	
Group	A	16	39	55
	B	39	106	145
		55	145	200

Expected		Outcome		
		Yes	No	
Group	A	15.125	39.875	55
	B	39.875	105.125	145
		55	145	200

Parameter	PE	SE	95%	IE
p(Yes|A)	0.290909	0.061242	0.170875	0.410943
p(Yes|B)	0.268966	0.036824	0.19679	0.341141
Probability Difference	0.021944	0.07146	−0.11812	0.162006
Probability Ratio	1.081585	0.251123	0.661151	1.769378
Odds Ratio	1.115056	0.351021	0.560404	2.218667

Test	Chi-Sq	p
Pearson's (uncorrected)	0.096304	0.756311
Pearson's (corrected)	0.017689	0.894195
Mantel-Haenszel	0.095823	0.756902
Fisher's Exact		1

Summary Estimates

Probability Ratio	
M-H Numerator	11.6
M-H Denominator	10.725
Weight	15.85725

Odds Ratio	
M-H Numerator	8.48
M-H Denominator	7.605
Weight	8.115828

Summary Chi-Square	
Observed	16
Expected	15.125
Variance	7.990028

The probability difference is 0.0219, the probability ratio is 1.0816, and the odds ratio is 1.1151.

Imagine we are interested in studying this relationship so we can better understand the etiology of CAD. That being the case, we would prefer to use either the probability ratio or odds ratio to summarize the relationship between diabetes and CAD. In the rest of this example, we will use the odds ratio.

Now, let us turn this into a multivariable data set by adding another independent variable. Suppose we want to control for smoking. In stratified analysis, additional nominal independent variables are used to create "strata." To control for smoking, we divide the data into one stratum in which everybody smokes and another stratum in which nobody smokes:

Smokers		CAD			Nonsmokers		CAD		
		YES	NO				YES	NO	
Diabetes	YES	8	7	15	Diabetes	YES	8	32	40
	NO	16	19	35		NO	23	87	110

12.7. Determine an odds ratio for each of those strata. How can we interpret those odds ratios?

Observed		Outcome			Expected		Outcome		
		Yes	No				Yes	No	
Group	A	8	7	15	Group	A	7.2	7.8	15
	B	16	19	35		B	16.8	18.2	35
		24	26	50			24	26	50

Parameter	PE	SE	95%	IE
p(YesIA)	0.533333	0.128812	0.280861	0.785805
p(YesIB)	0.457143	0.084204	0.292102	0.622183
Probability Difference	0.07619	0.153893	−0.22544	0.37782
Probability Ratio	1.166667	0.303746	0.643269	2.115928
Odds Ratio	1.357143	0.618861	0.403497	4.564682

Test	Chi-Sq	P
Pearson's (uncorrected)	0.2442	0.621189
Pearson's (corrected)	0.034341	0.852984
Mantel-Haenszel	0.239316	0.6247
Fisher's Exact		0.759773

Summary Estimates

Probability Ratio		Odds Ratio		Summary Chi-Square	
M-H Numerator	5.6	M-H Numerator	3.04	Observed	8
M-H Denominator	4.8	M-H Denominator	2.24	Expected	7.2
Weight	10.83871	Weight	2.611043	Variance	2.674286

The odds ratio for smokers is 1.3571. This implies that smoking persons with diabetes have somewhat higher odds of developing CAD than do smoking persons without diabetes.

Observed		Outcome			Expected		Outcome		
		Yes	No				Yes	No	
Group	A	8	32	40	Group	A	10.66667	29.33333	40
	B	23	78	110		B	29.33333	80.66667	110
		40	110	150			40	110	150

Parameter	PE	SE	95%	IE
p(YesIA)	0.2	0.063246	0.076039	0.323961
p(YesIB)	0.209091	0.038773	0.133095	0.285087
Probability Difference	−0.00909	0.074185	−0.15449	0.136311
Probability Ratio	0.956522	0.366589	0.466281	1.962192
Odds Ratio	0.945652	0.45959	0.384168	2.32778

Test	Chi-Sq	P
Pearson's (uncorrected)	0.014786	0.903218
Pearson's (corrected)	0.011321	0.915267
Mantel-Haenszel	0.014687	0.903539
Fisher's Exact		1

Summary Estimates

Probability Ratio		Odds Ratio		Summary Chi-Square	
M-H Numerator	5.866667	M-H Numerator	4.64	Observed	8
M-H Denominator	6.133333	M-H Denominator	4.906667	Expected	8.266667
Weight	7.441176	Weight	4.734344	Variance	4.841641

The odds ratio for nonsmokers is 0.9457. This implies that nonsmoking persons with diabetes have slightly lower odds of developing CAD than do nonsmoking persons without diabetes.

12.8. Calculate the summary estimate of the odds ratio describing the association between diabetes and CAD. How can we interpret this odds ratio?

$$OR \triangleq \overline{OR} = \frac{\sum\limits_{i=1}^{k} a_i \cdot d_i \big/ n_i}{\sum\limits_{i=1}^{k} b_i \cdot c_i \big/ n_i} = \frac{3.04 + 4.64}{2.24 + 4.906667} = 1.075$$

The odds of CAD among diabetics is slightly greater (1.075 times the odds) in nondiabetics.

12.9. Does it make sense to report the summary odds ratio instead of the strata-specific odds ratios? Why?

$$\chi^2_{(k-1)df} = \sum\limits_{i=1}^{k} \frac{(OR_i - \overline{OR})^2}{\frac{1}{w_i}} = \frac{(1.357143 - 1.075)^2}{\frac{1}{2.611043}} + \frac{(0.956522 - 1.075)^2}{\frac{1}{4.734344}} = 0.274$$

Since 0.274 is less than 3.841, we fail to reject the null hypothesis. This implies it makes sense to report the summary estimate.

12.10. Perform a Mantel-Haenszel test of the null hypothesis that the odds ratio describing the association between diabetes and CAD is equal to one in the population.

$$\chi^2_{1df} = \frac{\left(\sum a_i - \sum \frac{(a_i + b_i) \cdot (a_i + c_i)}{n_i}\right)^2}{\sum \frac{(a_i + b_i) \cdot (c_i + d_i) \cdot (a_i + c_i) \cdot (b_i + d_i)}{n_i^2 \cdot (n_i - 1)}}$$

$$= \frac{((8+8) - (7.2 + 8.266667))^2}{2.674286 + 4.842641} = 0.038$$

Since 0.038 is less than 3.841, we fail to reject the null hypothesis.

Suppose we are interested in survival in two cohorts (A and B).

Table 12.2   Mortality experience for persons in cohort A.

Time	Persons	Deaths	Withdrawals
1	500	25	70
2	405	22	65
3	318	19	64
4	235	16	97
5	122	7	115

Table 12.3   Mortality experience for persons in cohort B.

Time	Persons	Deaths	Withdrawals
1	500	40	63
2	397	36	58
3	303	27	44
4	232	17	79
5	136	12	124

12.11. Complete those as Kaplan-Meir life tables.

Table 12.4   Life table showing survival experience for persons in cohort A.

Time	Persons	Deaths	Withdrawals	p(live)	Cumulative p
1	500	25	70	0.950	0.950
2	405	22	65	0.946	0.898
3	318	19	64	0.940	0.845
4	235	16	97	0.932	0.787
5	122	7	115	0.943	0.742

Table 12.5   Life table showing survival experience for persons in cohort B.

Time	Persons	Deaths	Withdrawals	p(live)	Cumulative p
1	500	40	63	0.920	0.920
2	397	36	58	0.909	0.837
3	303	27	44	0.911	0.762
4	232	17	79	0.927	0.706
5	136	12	124	0.912	0.634

12.12. Calculate the mortality ratio for the two cohorts. How do we interpret this mortality ratio?

$$MR = \frac{1 - 0.742}{1 - 0.634} = 0.705$$

The five-year risk of mortality (MR) in Cohort A is about two-thirds of that in Cohort B, using the Kaplan-Meier method.

12.13. Test the null hypothesis that the mortality ratio is equal to one in the population allowing a 5% chance of making a type I error. Interpret the result.

Time = 1

Observed		Outcome				Expected		Outcome			
		Yes	No					Yes	No		
Group	A	25	475	500		Group	A	32.5	467.5	500	
	B	40	460	500			B	32.5	467.5	500	
		65	935	1000				65	935	1000	

Parameter	PE	SE	95%	IE		Test	Chi-Sq	P
p(Yes|A)	0.05	0.009747	0.030896	0.069104		Pearson's (uncorrected)	3.70218	0.054341
p(Yes|B)	0.08	0.012133	0.05622	0.10378		Pearson's (corrected)	3.22501	0.072521
Probability Difference	-0.03	0.015563	-0.0605	0.000503		Mantel-Haenszel	3.698478	0.054462
Probability Ratio	0.625	0.246982	0.385163	1.01418		Fisher's Exact		0.055607
Odds Ratio	0.605263	0.263209	0.361323	1.013894				

Summary Estimates

Probability Ratio		Odds Ratio		Summary Chi-Square	
M-H Numerator	12.5	M-H Numerator	11.5	Observed	25
M-H Denominator	20	M-H Denominator	19	Expected	32.5
Weight	16.39344	Weight	14.43435	Variance	15.20896

Time = 2

Observed		Outcome				Expected		Outcome		
		Yes	No					Yes	No	
Group	A	22	383	405		Group	A	29.28928	375.7107	405
	B	36	361	397			B	28.71072	368.2893	397
		58	744	802				58	744	802

Parameter	PE	SE	95%	IE		Test	Chi-Sq	P
p(Yes|A)	0.054321	0.011262	0.032247	0.076395		Pearson's (uncorrected)	3.950441	0.046859
p(Yes|B)	0.09068	0.014412	0.062433	0.118927		Pearson's (corrected)	3.427076	0.064136
Probability Difference	-0.03636	0.01829	-0.07221	-0.00051		Mantel-Haenszel	3.945515	0.046996
Probability Ratio	0.59904	0.261236	0.358994	0.999596		Fisher's Exact		0.076474
Odds Ratio	0.576008	0.280381	0.332479	0.997915				

Summary Estimates

Probability Ratio		Odds Ratio		Summary Chi-Square	
M-H Numerator	10.89027	M-H Numerator	9.902743	Observed	22
M-H Denominator	18.17955	M-H Denominator	17.19202	Expected	29.28928
Weight	14.65324	Weight	12.72048	Variance	13.46682

Time = 3

Observed		Outcome		
		Yes	No	
Group	A	19	299	318
	B	27	276	303
		46	575	621

Expected		Outcome		
		Yes	No	
Group	A	23.55556	294.4444	318
	B	22.44444	280.5556	303
		46	575	621

Parameter	PE	SE	95%	IE
p(Yes|A)	0.059748	0.013291	0.033697	0.0858
p(Yes|B)	0.089109	0.016367	0.057029	0.121188
Probability Diff	−0.02936	0.021084	−0.07069	0.011965
Probability Ratio	0.67051	0.288485	0.380927	6.351993
Odds Ratio	0.649573	0.310864	0.353195	1.194649

Test	Chi-Sq	P-value
Pearson's (Uncorrected)	1.950123	0.162574
Pearson's (corrected)	1.545539	0.213795
Mantel-Haenszel	1.946983	0.162912
Fisher's Exact		0.171059

Summary Estimates

Probability Ratio	
M-H Numerator	9.270531
M-H Denominator	13.82609
Weight	12.01582

Odds Ratio	
M-H Numerator	8.444444
M-H Denominator	13
Weight	10.34808

Summary Chi-Square	
Observed	19
Expected	23.55556
Variance	10.6591

Time = 4

Observed		Outcome		
		Yes	No	
Group	A	16	219	235
	B	17	215	232
		33	434	467

Expected		Outcome		
		Yes	No	
Group	A	16.606	218.394	235
	B	16.394	215.606	232
		33	434	467

Parameter	PE	SE	95%	IE
p(Yes|A)	0.068085	0.016432	0.035879	0.100291
p(Yes|B)	0.073276	0.017108	0.039743	0.106809
Probability Diff	−0.00519	0.023721	−0.05168	0.041303
Probability Ratio	0.929161	0.335794	0.481124	9.228732
Odds Ratio	0.923986	0.361304	0.45511	1.875918

Test	Chi-Sq	P-value
Pearson's (Uncorrected)	0.047899	0.82676
Pearson's (corrected)	0.001465	0.969464
Mantel-Haenszel	0.047797	0.826942
Fisher's Exact		0.858394

Summary Estimates

Probability Ratio	
M-H Numerator	7.948608
M-H Denominator	8.554604
Weight	8.868561

Odds Ratio	
M-H Numerator	7.366167
M-H Denominator	7.972163
Weight	7.660434

Summary Chi-Square	
Observed	16
Expected	16.606
Variance	7.683159

Time = 5

Observed		Outcome		
		Yes	No	
Group	A	7	115	122
	B	12	124	136
		19	239	258

Expected		Outcome		
		Yes	No	
Group	A	8.984496	113.0155	122
	B	10.0155	125.9845	136
		19	239	258

Parameter	PE	SE	95%	IE
p(Yes|A)	0.057377	0.021055	0.016109	0.098645
p(Yes|B)	0.088235	0.024322	0.040565	0.135906
Probability Diff	−0.03086	0.032169	−0.09391	0.032194
Probability Ratio	0.650273	0.458956	0.264499	7.305252
Odds Ratio	0.628986	0.4929	0.239373	1.652745

Test	Chi-Sq	P-value
Pearson's (Uncorrected)	0.897655	0.343411
Pearson's (corrected)	0.502304	0.478489
Mantel-Haenszel	0.894176	0.344348
Fisher's Exact		0.474902

Summary Estimates

Probability Ratio	
M-H Numerator	3.689922
M-H Denominator	5.674419
Weight	4.747418

Odds Ratio	
M-H Numerator	3.364341
M-H Denominator	5.348837
Weight	4.116062

Summary Chi-Square	
Observed	7
Expected	8.984496
Variance	4.404308

$$\chi^2_{1df} = \frac{\left(\sum a_i - \sum \frac{(a_i + b_i)\cdot(a_i + c_i)}{n_i}\right)^2}{\sum \frac{(a_i + b_i)\cdot(c_i + d_i)\cdot(a_i + c_i)\cdot(b_i + d_i)}{n_i^2 \cdot (n_i - 1)}} = \frac{(89 - 10.94)^2}{51.422} = 9.361$$

This is greater than the critical value (3.841), so we reject the null hypothesis.

12.14. Use the "Life Table" BAHR program to analyze these data.

An easier way to analyze these data is with the "Life Table Analysis" BAHR program. Those results follow:

Life Table Analysis

What is the name of this group?

Cohort A

Time	Number	Events	Withdrawals	p(t)	p(T)
1	500	25	70	0.950	0.950
2	405	22	65	0.946	0.898
3	318	19	64	0.940	0.845
4	235	16	97	0.932	0.787
5	122	7	115	0.943	0.742

Next

Life Table Analysis

What is the name of this group?

Cohort B

Time	Number	Events	Withdrawals	p(t)	p(T)
1	500	40	63	0.920	0.920
2	397	36	58	0.909	0.837
3	303	27	44	0.911	0.762
4	232	17	79	0.927	0.706
5	136	12	124	0.912	0.634

Next

	Cumulative Risks			95% Interval Est.	
Time	Cohort A	Cohort B	Risk Ratio	LL	UL
1	0.05	0.08	0.625	1.009048	0.387122
2	0.101605	0.163426	0.621719	0.87112	0.443722
3	0.155283	0.237972	0.652525	0.855876	0.497489
4	0.212795	0.29381	0.724261	0.900068	0.582794
5	0.257963	0.356121	0.724368	0.890616	0.589154

We can use this table in the output to test the null hypothesis that the risk ratio for a period of time is equal to one with α equal to 0.05 by examining the confidence intervals. For example, the confidence interval for the five-year risk excludes one. Thus, we can conclude that there is a statistically significant risk ratio for five-year risks. This corresponds to the results when we tested this null hypothesis manually.

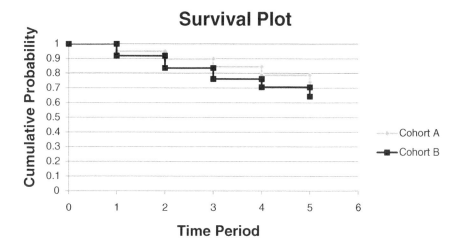

The survival plot provided to us by the "Life Table" BAHR program gives us the impression that the cumulative probability (the complement of risk) for Cohort B is consistently lower than the cumulative probability for Cohort A. That difference is not large, but it is consistent. It is sufficiently large to allow us to reject null hypotheses about the two-year risk, three-year risk, and four-year risk as well as the five-year risk (Example 12.13).

EXERCISES

12.1. The Framingham Heart Study (FHS) focused on risk factors for heart disease. Suppose we want to compare the odds of getting heart disease for age, gender (sex = 1 for men, sex = 0 for women), serum cholesterol (scl), diastolic blood pressure (dbp), and body mass index (bmi). We include age and gender to control for their effect. The data for the first 500 persons participating in the FHS is in the Excel file: EXR12_1. Perform a logistic regression analysis on those data with an indicator of heart disease as the dependent variable. From that analysis, do you think the relationship between BMI and heart disease is different for men compared to women?

   A. No, they are the same

   B. Yes, but they are not significantly different

   C. Yes, and they are significantly different

12.2. The Framingham Heart Study (FHS) focused on risk factors for heart disease. Suppose we want to compare the odds of getting heart disease for age, gender (sex = 1 for men, sex = 0 for women), serum cholesterol (scl), diastolic blood pressure (dbp), and body mass index (bmi). We include age and gender to control for their effect. The data for the first 500 persons participating in the FHS is in the Excel file: EXR12_1. Perform a logistic regression analysis on those data with an indicator of heart disease as the dependent variable. From that analysis, do you think the intercepts of the regression lines for men and women are different?

A. No, they are the same

B. Yes, but they are not significantly different

C. Yes, and they are significantly different

12.3. The Framingham Heart Study (FHS) focused on risk factors for heart disease. Suppose we want to compare the odds of getting heart disease for age, gender (sex = 1 for men, sex = 0 for women), serum cholesterol (scl), diastolic blood pressure (dbp), and body mass index (bmi). We include age and gender to control for their effect. The data for the first 500 persons participating in the FHS is in the Excel file: EXR12_1. Perform a logistic regression analysis on those data with an indicator of heart disease as the dependent variable. From that analysis, which independent variables are independent risk factors? Select as many as there are correct answers.

A. Serum cholesterol

B. Body mass index

C. Diastolic blood pressure

12.4. The Framingham Heart Study (FHS) focused on risk factors for heart disease. Suppose we want to compare the odds of getting heart disease for age, gender (sex = 1 for men, sex = 0 for women), serum cholesterol (scl), diastolic blood pressure (dbp), and body mass index (bmi). We include age and gender to control for their effect. The data for the first 500 persons participating in the FHS is in the Excel file: EXR12_1. Perform a logistic regression analysis on those data with an indicator of heart disease as the dependent variable. From that analysis, estimate the odds ratio of heart disease for a five year difference in age. Which of the following is closest to that odds ratio?

A. 1.00

B. 1.20

C. 1.33

D. 2.00

E. 2.66

12.5. The Framingham Heart Study (FHS) focused on risk factors for heart disease. Suppose we want to compare the odds of getting heart disease for age, gender (sex = 1 for men, sex = 0 for women), serum cholesterol (scl), diastolic blood pressure (dbp), and body mass index (bmi). We include age and gender to control for their effect. The data for the first 500 persons participating in the FHS is in the Excel file: EXR12_1. Perform a logistic regression analysis on those data with an indicator of heart disease as the dependent variable. From that analysis, estimate the odds ratio of heart disease for a two-unit difference in BMI among women. Which of the following is closest to that odds ratio?

A. 1.00

B. 1.20

C. 1.33

D. 2.00

E. 2.66

12.6. Suppose we were to conduct a case-control study to investigate the relationship between exposure to dust produced by a particular industry and development of chronic obstructive pulmonary disease (COPD). Also suppose that we want to control for smoking as a potential confounder. For smokers, 25 out of 50 cases and 10 out of 50 controls were exposed. For nonsmokers, 15 out of 50 cases and six out of 50 controls were exposed. Determine the summary odds ratio for those data. Which of the following is closest to your answer?

A. 2.44

B. 2.89

C. 3.22

D. 3.61

E. 3.74

12.7. Suppose we were to conduct a cohort study to investigate the relationship between exposure to cigarette smoke and development of cataracts. Also suppose that we want to control for gender as a potential confounder. For men, 12 out of 50 exposed and four out of 50 unexposed persons developed cataracts. For women, eight out of 50 exposed and seven out of 50 unexposed persons developed cataracts. Calculate the summary probability ratio for those data. Which of the following is closest to your answer?

A. 1.14

B. 1.82

C. 2.63

D. 3.00

E. 3.22

12.8. Suppose we were to conduct a case-control study to investigate the relationship between exposure to dust produced by a particular industry and development of chronic obstructive pulmonary disease (COPD). Also suppose that we want to control for smoking as a potential confounder. For smokers, 25 out of 50 cases and 10 out of 50 controls were exposed. For nonsmokers, 15 out of 50 cases and six out of 50 controls were exposed. Does it make sense to report the summary odds ratio for those data?

A. No, since the strata-specific odds ratios are too different

B. Yes, since the strata-specific odds ratios are not too different

C. Yes, because the test of homogeneity is significant

D. Yes, because the test of homogeneity is not significant

E. No, because the test of homogeneity is significant

F. No, because the test of homogeneity is not significant

12.9. Suppose we were to conduct a cohort study to investigate the relationship between exposure to cigarette smoke and development of cataracts. Also suppose that we want to control for gender as a potential confounder. For men, 12 out of 50 exposed and four out of 50 unexposed persons developed cataracts. For women, eight out of 50 exposed and seven out of 50 unexposed persons developed cataracts. Test the null hypothesis that the probability ratio is the same among men and women in the population. Which of the following is the best conclusion to draw?

A. Reject both the null and alternative hypotheses

B. Accept both the null and alternative hypotheses

C. Reject the null hypothesis and accept the alternative hypothesis

D. Accept the null hypothesis and reject the alternative hypothesis

E. It is best not to draw a conclusion about the null and alternative hypotheses from these data

12.10. Suppose we were to conduct a case-control study to investigate the relationship between exposure to dust produced by a particular industry and development of chronic obstructive pulmonary disease (COPD). Also suppose that we want to control for smoking as a potential confounder. For smokers, 25 out of 50 cases and 10 out of 50 controls were exposed. For nonsmokers, 15 out of 50 cases and six out of 50 controls were exposed. Test the null hypothesis that the odds ratio for exposure is equal to one in the population versus the alternative that is not equal to one, allowing a 5% chance of making a type I error. Which of the following is the best conclusion to draw?

A. Reject both the null and alternative hypotheses

B. Accept both the null and alternative hypotheses

C. Reject the null hypothesis and accept the alternative hypothesis

D. Accept the null hypothesis and reject the alternative hypothesis

E. It is best not to draw a conclusion about the null and alternative hypotheses from these data

12.11. Suppose we investigate the rate of cure over a three-week period among persons who received a new treatment for Lyme disease. These data are in the Excel file: EXR12_2. What is the probability that a person who receives the new treatment will be cured within three weeks?

A. 0.40

B. 0.49

C. 0.51

D. 0.55

E. 0.60

12.12. Suppose we investigate a new treatment for a particular type of breast cancer by comparing it to the standard treatment in 400 women with stage III breast cancer. The survival over five years appears in the Excel file: EXR12_3. What is the five-year risk of fatality among patients who received the standard treatment?

A. 0.24

B. 0.31

C. 0.36

D. 0.44

E. 0.65

12.13. Suppose we investigate the rate of cure over a three-week period among persons who received a new treatment for Lyme disease and among persons who received the standard treatment. These data are in the Excel file: EXR12_2. What is the probability ratio comparing persons who received the new treatment to persons who received the standard treatment?

A. 1.80

B. 2.00

C. 2.33

D. 3.15

E. 4.36

12.14. Suppose we investigate a new treatment for a particular type of breast cancer by comparing it to the standard treatment in 400 women with stage III breast cancer. The survival over five years appears in the Excel file: EXR12_3. What is the five-year probability ratio comparing persons who received the new treatment to persons who received the standard treatment?

A. 1.24

B. 2.19

C. 2.57

D. 2.86

E. 3.22

12.15. Suppose we investigate the rate of cure over a 3-week period among persons who received a new treatment for Lyme disease and among persons who received the standard treatment. These data are in the Excel file: EXR12_2. Test the null hypothesis that the three-year probability ratio is equal to one in the population versus the alternative that is not equal to one allowing a 5% chance of making a type I error. Which of the following is the best conclusion to draw?

A. Reject both the null and alternative hypotheses

B. Accept both the null and alternative hypotheses

C. Reject the null hypothesis and accept the alternative hypothesis

D. Accept the null hypothesis and reject the alternative hypothesis

E. It is best not to draw a conclusion about the null and alternative hypotheses from these data

12.16. Suppose we investigate a new treatment for a particular type of breast cancer by comparing it to the standard treatment in 400 women with stage III breast cancer. The survival over five years appears in the Excel file: EXR12_3. Test the null hypothesis that the five-year probability ratio is equal to one in the population versus the alternative that is not equal to one allowing a 5% chance of making a type I error. Which of the following is the best conclusion to draw?

A. Reject both the null and alternative hypotheses

B. Accept both the null and alternative hypotheses

C. Reject the null hypothesis and accept the alternative hypothesis

D. Accept the null hypothesis and reject the alternative hypothesis

E. It is best not to draw a conclusion about the null and alternative hypotheses from these data

CHAPTER 13

Selecting Statistical Tests

OVERVIEW

The last nine chapters of the textbook are structured around flowcharts that describe how a statistician selects a method of analysis for a particular dataset and a particular research question. While reading each of those chapters, the flowcharts gave us an idea about how the statistical procedures described fit into the organization of statistical methods, but we were focused on the methods being described rather than the overall structure of the flowcharts. Chapter 13 in the workbook gives us an opportunity to step back and consider the all of flowcharts.

The flowcharts are collected in Appendix A of both the textbook and the workbook, as well as at the beginning of each of the last nine chapters of the textbook. To start, consider the master flowchart (Flowchart 1). This is where we begin to select an appropriate approach to a set of data. First, we need to identify the dependent variable. We can do this by asking ourselves, "What do we want to

Workbook to Accompany Introduction to Biostatistical Applications in Health Research with Microsoft® Office Excel®, First Edition. Robert P. Hirsch.
© 2016 John Wiley & Sons, Inc. Published 2016 by John Wiley & Sons, Inc.

make an estimate of or test a hypothesis about?" The answer is the dependent variable. It is not unusual to have more than one dependent variable in a dataset. That is ok. The most common approach to this situation is to consider each of the dependent variables, one at a time.

Next, we need to identify the independent variable(s). We find these by asking ourselves, "Under what conditions are we interested in examining the dependent variable?" For example, this could be comparing groups of dependent variable values. Nominal independent variables are needed to specify these groups. We need one fewer nominal independent variable(s) than there are groups to compare. Our concern at this point is just to count the independent variables and decide if there are no independent variables, one independent variable, or more than one independent variable.

The final thing we need to do with the master flowchart (Flowchart 1) is decide what type of data is being represented by the dependent variable. We need to choose among three types: continuous, ordinal, or nominal. The introduction to Part Two in the textbook describes these types of data. To summarize, the types of data differ according to their ability to order the data values in a biologically meaningful way and according to the spacing between values. Continuous data have ordered, evenly-spaced values. Ordinal data have ordered values, but the spacing between values is undefined. Nominal data cannot be ordered in a meaningful way. Identifying the type of data represented by the dependent variable gets us to the next part of the flowchart, each associated with a chapter of the textbook.

The next thing we do depends on whether or not there are independent variables. If there are independent variables, we need to identify the type of data represented by those independent variables. Then, we might have committed to a single path to the end of the flowchart, or there may be more decisions to make. These decisions are related to the research interest, and the nature of the independent variable(s).

As we approach the end of the flowchart, three pieces of information are itemized. First, there is the point estimate(s) that is most often of interest. Next comes the common name of the procedure. Finally, there is the name of the general method or standard distribution that is used to perform the analysis. Now, we know quite a bit about how to analyze a particular set of data, but there still might be decisions to make. For example, we need to decide whether we want to take chance into account by calculating an interval estimate or by hypothesis testing. We turn to Chapter 3 of the textbook to answer that question. Other decisions are discussed in the chapter to which the flowchart belongs.

GLOSSARY

Bivariable Dataset – a collection of data that includes one dependent variable and one independent variable.

Continuous Data – measurements that can be ordered and that are evenly-spaced. They generally have a large number of possible values.

Dependent Variable – the variable that represents the data of primary interest. These are the data for which we want to make an estimate or test a hypothesis.

Independent Variable – a variable that represents data that specify conditions under which we are interested in the dependent variable.

Multivariable Dataset – a collection of data that includes one dependent variable and more than one independent variable.

Multivariate Methods – statistical methods designed to analyze more than one dependent variable in a single analysis. Multivariate methods are not commonly used in health research.

Nominal Data – measurements that cannot be ordered in a biologically meaningful way.

Ordinal Data – measurements that can be ordered, but where the spacing between values is uneven or undefined.

Univariable Dataset – a collection of data in which there is one dependent variable and no independent variables.

Variable – a theoretical entity that represents data in the mathematics of statistical methods.

EXAMPLES

13.1. A state health department has conducted a survey in a random sample of 500 high school students to estimate the frequency of two risk-taking behaviors: smoking and unprotected sexual intercourse. Among those persons in the sample, they found that 123 students were currently smoking and 97 students were regularly engaged in unprotected sexual intercourse. What type of point estimate should be used to summarize these observations?

We begin by trying to identify the data that will be represented by a dependent variable. We do this by asking ourselves for which data are we interested in making an estimate or testing a hypothesis. There are two types of data mentioned in this study: smoking and unprotected intercourse. We are equally interested in both, so there are two dependent variables. The usual biostatistical practice is to perform a separate analysis for each dependent variable. Thus, we consider the data in this example to be part of two, separate datasets. There are no specific conditions under which we are interested in examining these two dependent variables, so they are univariable datasets.

Both dependent variables represent nominal data. This means that Chapter 6 discusses how to analyze these data. There are three point estimates addressed in Chapter 6: prevalence, risk, and incidence. Incidence and risk address intervals of time. We do not have information on intervals of time; only a point in time. Therefore, we would estimate prevalences.

13.2. For the survey described in Example 13.1, what is the best way to take into account the role of chance in obtaining the sample of 500 students?

There are two aspects of taking chance into account that we need to consider. The first involves choosing between interval estimation and hypothesis testing. We can always perform interval estimation, but hypothesis testing requires a sensible (ie, of biologic interest) null hypothesis. When we have a univariable dataset, a sensible null hypothesis requires a paired sample. This is not a paired sample, so we will use interval estimation.

The second aspect is particular to nominal dependent variables. It is the choice between an exact procedure and a normal approximation. The better choice is the exact procedure, if we have a computer program to perform it. Otherwise, the normal approximation is the better choice.

13.3. A group of researchers is studying the relationship between RBC (red blood cell) counts and doses of folic acid. In this study, they randomly assign 100 persons with pernicious anemia to each of 10 doses of folic acid and, after a period of two weeks, they perform a RBC count. What point estimate(s) should they use to summarize these observations?

Here we have two types of data: RBC counts and dose of folic acid. When we ask ourselves which we want to make estimates of, the answer is RBC counts. Dose specifies the condition under which we are in interested in RBC counts. Thus, it is represented by an independent variable. It is the only independent variable, so we have a bivariable dataset. The dependent variable is RBC counts which can be considered continuous, so, we are interested in the flowchart in Chapter 7.

Now that we have an independent variable, the next thing we need to decide is what type of data are represented by the independent variable. Doses are continuous, so we are in the left-hand branch of the flowchart. Now, we have to decide what question the researchers are asking. Do they want to estimate RBC for a given dose or do they want to describe the strength of the association between RBC and dose? This is not completely clear, but the likely answer is that they want to describe the relationship, rather than say how strong it is. Thus, "Intercept and slope" is the best answer.

13.4. In the study described in Example 13.3, the researchers are concerned about potential confounding effects of gender in their investigation of the relationship between RBC counts and dose of folic acid. What is the name of the general class of statistical procedures that they should use to analyze these observations while controlling for gender?

This is a continuation of Example 13.3. What has changed is that another variable has been established. This is gender. The interest in including gender is to control for its effect. Thus, gender is represented by an independent variable. Now, we have two independent variables: dose and gender. This means we have a multivariable dataset with a continuous dependent variable. This puts us in Chapter 10 of the textbook. Since we have both a continuous (dose) and a nominal (gender) independent variable, we find ourselves in the right-hand branch of the flowchart. This leads to analysis of covariance.

13.5. Suppose we conducted a study of serum cholesterol levels among persons randomly sampled from five different countries. In the analysis of these data, we are interested in comparing mean serum cholesterol levels between genders as well as between countries. What is the name of the general class of statistical procedures that we should use to analyze these data?

In this study, it is clear that serum cholesterol is represented by the dependent variable and that gender and country will be represented by independent variables. We have more than one independent variable and the dependent variable is continuous, so we are in Chapter 10 of the textbook. All independent variables are nominal, so we are in the middle branch of the flowchart. Here, we have to decide whether the nominal independent variables specify categories of one or more than one characteristic. There are two characteristics: gender and country. Thus, we want to use a factorial analysis of variance to analyze these data.

13.6. Suppose we are interested in the strength of the relationship between body mass index (BMI) and systolic blood pressure (SBP). To investigate this relationship, we randomly select 250 persons from a particular population and measure their BMI and SBP. What point estimate(s) would be the most appropriate to summarize the data?

It is not clear which of the two continuous variables is the dependent variable and which is the independent variable. That often is the case when the interest is in the strength of the association between two continuous variables. That does not impede our use of the flowchart. It is clear that the dependent variable must be continuous and that we have one independent variable. Thus, we are in Chapter 7 of the textbook. The independent variable is continuous, so we are in the left-hand branch of that flowchart. If we follow the path for strength of the association, we encounter Pearson's correlation coefficient.

13.7. For the data in Example 13.6, suppose we are interested in estimating the mean SBP for persons with a particular BMI. What point estimates would be the most appropriate to summarize the data to reflect that interest?

This is a modification of Example 13.6. Now we know the dependent variable represents SBP. The difference here, is the question being asked. Instead of strength of the association, we are interested in estimating dependent variable values corresponding to values of the independent variable. Thus, we take the branch that leads to slope and intercept.

13.8. What is the common name of the statistical method that would be best used to address the interest in Example 13.7?

This continuation of Example 13.7 requires us to follow the same branch of the flowchart so we can find the common name of the procedure. That name is linear regression analysis.

13.9. Now, suppose we want to control for age in the analysis addressing the interest described in Example 13.8. What is the common name of the statistical method that would be the best to use?

This is a continuation of Example 13.8. Here, we add a second continuous independent variable (age). That means we have a multivariable dataset. Since the dependent variable is continuous, we are in Chapter 10. Both independent variables are continuous, so we are in the left-hand branch of the flowchart. Our interest still is in estimating dependent variable values; thus we want to use multiple regression analysis.

13.10. Finally, suppose we want to control for both age and gender in the analysis addressing the interest described in Example 13.8. What is the common name of the statistical method that would be the best to use?

This is a continuation of Example 13.9. Gender is added as another independent variable. That means we have a mixture of continuous and nominal independent variables. This leads us to analysis of covariance.

13.11. Suppose we measure the serum cholesterol level for 50 persons on a particular diet. What is the best way to summarize those measurements while taking chance into account?

This is similar to Example 13.1 in that we need to decide between interval estimation and hypothesis testing as ways to take chance into account. As in Example 13.1, there is no sensible null hypothesis to test, so the only possible answer is interval estimation. If we were uncertain about what parameter to estimate, we could recognize this as a univariable sample with a continuous dependent variable. That selects the Chapter 4 flowchart.

13.12. For the study described in Example 13.11, suppose we want to look at how much the serum cholesterol changes when people use a particular diet. To study that change, we measure, for each of the 50 persons, serum cholesterol just prior to starting the diet and then again after being on the diet for 30 days. (i.e., both measurements are made for each individual person). What would be the best statistical test to analyze these data?

Here, we have two measurements of serum cholesterol for each person. We are told, however, it is neither measurement of serum cholesterol that is of interest. Instead the difference between the two measurements is the dependent variable. There are no other variables, so this is a univariable sample with a continuous dependent variable. That selects the flowchart in Chapter 4.

13.13. For the study described in Example 13.12, suppose we want to look at how strong the association is between serum cholesterol measured just prior to beginning the diet and after 30 days on the diet. To examine the strength of that association, what would be the best statistical test to use?

Although these are the same data as in Example 13.12, the question being asked changes how we think about those data. Instead of using the two measurements of serum cholesterol to find the difference, we are now interested in the two measurements themselves. Thus, this is a bivariable sample with a continuous dependent variable. This puts us in Chapter 7. There, we are in the left-hand branch because the independent variable represents continuous data as well. We are interested in the strength of association, so we follow the flowchart to Pearson's correlation coefficient.

13.14. For the study described in Example 13.12, suppose there are actually three diets of interest to us and that we randomly assign 50 different persons to each of them. To compare the mean change in serum cholesterol among those three diets, what would be the best statistical test to use?

This is a continuation of Example 13.12 in which the difference between cholesterol measurements is the dependent variable. Now, we are going to divide those differences into three groups. To specify three groups of dependent variable values, we need two nominal independent variables.[1] Thus, we have a multivariable sample with a continuous dependent variable. This puts us in Chapter 10.

---

[1] Recall that nominal variables are dichotomous, so it takes k-1 nominal variables to specify k groups.

Both of the independent variables represent nominal data, so we are in the middle branch of the flowchart. Diet is a single characteristic. This leads us to one-way analysis of variance.

13.15. For the study described in Example 13.14, suppose we are also interested in the ability of chitosan to reduce the serum cholesterol further. To study this treatment, we randomly assign each of the 50 persons on each diet to receive either chitosan or a placebo. To look at the effect of chitosan as well as the effect of the diets, what would be the best statistical test to analyze these data?

This is a continuation of Example 13.14. Now, we are adding another treatment to diet. This creates six groups of dependent variable values, so we have five nominal independent variables. This keeps us in the middle branch of the flowchart. When we changed the number of groups to six, we also added another characteristic (chitosan). Thus, the flowchart leads us to factorial analysis of variance.

13.16. For the study described in Example 13.15, suppose we want to compare serum cholesterol values for the three diets and two treatments while controlling for the potential confounding of age and gender. What would be the best statistical test to analyze these data?

This is a continuation of Example 13.15. We have added two more independent variables: gender and age. Since we now have both nominal and continuous independent variables, we are in the right-hand branch of the flowchart in Chapter 10. This branch leads to analysis of covariance.

13.17. Imagine we are interested in the relationship between HPV (human papilloma virus) and development of cervical cancer. To study this relationship, we identify 1,000 women with normal PAP smears who are positive for HPV and follow them for five years. During that period, each of the women receive biannual examinations, including a PAP smear. Of those 1,000 women, 250 of them develop abnormal PAP smears during the five-year period. What would be the best point estimate to summarize those results?

The dependent variable represents developing an abnormal PAP smear. This is a nominal dependent variable. There are no independent variables.[2] This means we have a univariable sample with a nominal dependent variable. This puts us in Chapter 6. In the Chapter 6 flowchart we need to distinguish between a nominal dependent variable affected by time and not affected by time. Since everyone was

---

[2] HPV is a constant, not a variable. Everyone was positive for HPV.

followed for a five-year period, the dependent variable is not affected by time. This means we can estimate a probability. There are three probabilities listed among the answers. Since we are interested in new cases developed over time, it is the five-year risk we want to estimate.

13.18. Now, suppose we identify another 1,000 women with normal PAP smears who are negative for HPV and we follow these women for five years as well. During that period of time, 75 of these 1,000 women develop abnormal PAP smears. What is the best point estimate to compare the results for these women to the results for the women in Example 13.17 if we do not want the comparison to reflect the underlying frequency of abnormal PAP smears?

This is a continuation of Example 13.17. Another group of women is added to the study. Now, HPV is an independent variable. This means we have a bivariable sample with a nominal dependent variable. We are in Chapter 9. Since HPV is a nominal variable, we follow the right-hand branch of the flowchart. As explained in Example 13.14, the dependent variable is not affected by time. Since there is no attempt to pair HPV persons to non-HPV persons, this is an unpaired study. This leads us to a choice among three parameters to estimate. To make this choice, we recall from Chapter 6 that ratios are not affected by the underlying frequency of the event or characteristic.

13.19. For the study described in Examples 13.17 and 13.18, what is the common name of the statistical method that would be best to test a null hypothesis about the occurrence of abnormal PAP smears between the two groups of women?

This is a continuation of Example 13.18. Now, we are to continue down the flowchart to find the common name of the statistical method we should use. There are two: a normal approximation and an exact test. We learned in Chapter 6 that, if we have a choice, we should use the results from the exact test.

EXERCISES

13.1. Suppose we are interested in how well a new medication prevents migraine headaches. To study this relationship, we identify 200 persons who suffer from migraines. Then, we assign 100 people to receive the new medication and 100 people to receive the standard therapy and record the number of people who have at least one migraine during a three-month period. In this study, the dependent variable represents which of the following?

   A. People in the population

   B. People with a history of migraines

    C. Occurrence of migraine during the three-month study period

    D. The new medication

    E. The distinction between the new medication and the standard therapy

13.2. Suppose we measure the diastolic blood pressure for 25 students taking this examination. Which of the following is the best way to summarize those measurements?

    A. Estimate the mean diastolic blood pressure and calculate its 95% confidence interval

    B. Estimate the mean diastolic blood pressure and test the null hypothesis that it is equal to zero in the population

    C. Estimate the proportion of persons with high blood pressure and test the null hypothesis that it is equal to zero in the population

    D. Estimate the proportion of persons with high blood pressure and test the null hypothesis that it is equal to 0.5 in the population

    E. Estimate the proportion of persons with high blood pressure and test the null hypothesis that it is equal to one in the population

13.3. Suppose we measure the diastolic blood pressure for 25 students taking this examination. Further suppose we want to look at how much diastolic blood pressure changes between the last lecture and the final examination. To examine that change, we measure for each of the 25 students diastolic blood pressure both during the last lecture and the final examination (i.e., both measurements are made for each individual student). Which of the following would be the best statistical test to analyze these data?

    A. Paired *t* test

    B. Student's *t* test

    C. Linear regression analysis

    D. Pearson's correlation analysis

    E. Normal approximation to the binomial

13.4. Suppose we measure the diastolic blood pressure for 25 students taking this examination. Further suppose we want to look at how much diastolic blood pressure changes between the last lecture and the final examination. To examine that change, we measure for each of the 25 students diastolic blood pressure both during the last lecture and the final examination (i.e., both measurements are made for each individual student). Now suppose we want to look at how strong the association is between diastolic blood pressure measured during the last lecture and diastolic blood pressure measured during the final examination. To examine the strength of that association, which of the following would be the best statistical test to use?

    A. Paired *t* test

    B. Student's *t* test

C. Linear regression analysis

D. Pearson's correlation analysis

E. Normal approximation to the binomial

13.5. Suppose we measure the diastolic blood pressure for 25 students taking this examination. Further suppose we want to look at how much diastolic blood pressure changes between the last lecture and the final examination. To examine that change, we measure for each of the 25 students diastolic blood pressure both during the last lecture and the final examination (i.e., both measurements are made for each individual student). Now, suppose that we want to compare diastolic blood pressure values during the final examination among students taking a statistics course during different semesters. Suppose that we measure diastolic blood pressure during the final for samples of 25 students for each of the three semesters (i.e., fall, spring, and summer) of one academic year. Which of the following would be the best statistical test to analyze these data?

A. Multiple regression analysis

B. Multiple correlation analysis

C. One-way analysis of variance

D. Factorial analysis of variance

E. Analysis of covariance

13.6. Suppose we measure the diastolic blood pressure for 25 students taking this examination. Further suppose we want to look at how much diastolic blood pressure changes between the last lecture and the final examination. To examine that change, we measure for each of the 25 students diastolic blood pressure both during the last lecture and the final examination (i.e., both measurements are made for each individual student). Now, suppose we want to compare diastolic blood pressure values during the final examination among students taking a statistics course during two different academic years (e.g., 2015-2016 and 2016-2017) as well as during different semesters in each of those years. Suppose that we measure diastolic blood pressure during the final for samples of 25 students for each of the three semesters (i.e., fall, spring, and summer) of each academic year. Which of the following would be the best statistical test to analyze these data?

A. Multiple regression analysis

B. Multiple correlation analysis

C. One-way analysis of variance

D. Factorial analysis of variance

E. Analysis of covariance

13.7. Suppose we measure the diastolic blood pressure for 25 students taking this examination. Further suppose we want to look at how much diastolic blood pressure changes between the last lecture and the final examination. To examine that change, we measure for each of the 25 students diastolic blood pressure both during the last lecture and the final examination (i.e., both measurements are made for each individual student). Now, suppose we want to compare diastolic blood pressure values during the final examination while controlling for the potential confounding of age and gender. Which of the following would be the best statistical test to analyze these data?

A. Multiple regression analysis

B. Multiple correlation analysis

C. One-way analysis of variance

D. Factorial analysis of variance

E. Analysis of covariance

13.8. Suppose that we are interested in the relationship between smoking and getting an "A" on a final examination. To study this relationship, we identify 25 smokers and 25 nonsmokers in a particular course. Then we determine how many in each of those groups got "A"s. Which of the following would be the best way to analyze those data?

A. Normal approximation to the binomial

B. Student's t test

C. Chi-square test

D. Logistic regression analysis

E. Multiple regression analysis

13.9. Suppose that we are interested in the relationship between smoking and getting an "A" on a final examination. To study this relationship, we identify 25 smokers and 25 nonsmokers in a particular course. Then we determine how many students in each of those groups got "A"s. Further suppose we want to control for age and gender. Which of the following would be the best way to analyze those data while controlling for these potential confounders?

A. Normal approximation to the binomial

B. Student's t test

C. Chi-square test

D. Logistic regression analysis

E. Multiple regression analysis

13.10. Suppose that we are interested in the change in heart rate that occurs during a particular form of exercise. To investigate this change, we select 100 persons to be in a study. In that study, each of the 100 persons have their heart rate measured before and, then, during exercise. Which of the following would be the best point estimate(s) to reflect this change?

A. Coefficient of determination

B. Mean of the differences in heart rates

    C. Difference between the mean heart rates

    D. Correlation coefficient

    E. Intercept and slope

13.11. Suppose that we are interested in the change in heart rate that occurs during a particular form of exercise. To investigate this change, we select 100 persons to be in a study. In that study, each of the 100 persons have their heart rate measured before and, then, during exercise. Now, suppose we are interested in estimating the heart rate during exercise based on an individual's heart rate before exercise while controlling for differences in heart rate related to body mass index (BMI). Which of the following is the common name of the statistical test that would be best to use in that analysis?

    A. Analysis of covariance

    B. Multiple regression analysis

    C. Student-Newman-Keuls test

    D. One-way analysis of variance

    E. Factorial analysis of variance

13.12. Suppose that we are interested in the change in heart rate that occurs during a particular form of exercise. To investigate this change, we select 100 persons to be in a study. In that study, each of the 100 persons have their heart rate measured before and, then, during exercise. Now, suppose we are interested in estimating the heart rate during exercise based on an individual's heart rate before exercise while controlling for differences in heart rate related to body mass index (BMI) and gender. Which of the following is the common name of the statistical test that would be best to use in that analysis?

    A. Analysis of covariance

    B. Multiple regression analysis

    C. Student-Newman-Keuls test

    D. One-way analysis of variance

    E. Factorial analysis of variance

13.13. Suppose that we are interested in studying the association between being exposed to second-hand smoke and having a low birth-weight infant. To study this association, we identify 50 women who have recently delivered a singleton infant and who were exposed to second-hand smoke during their pregnancy and 50 women who have recently delivered a singleton infant and who were not exposed to second-hand smoke during their pregnancy. For each of these women we determine the birth-weight of their infant. Which of the following is the common name of the statistical procedure that would be best to use to compare birth-weights between these two groups of women?

    A. Fisher's exact test

    B. McNemar's test

    C. Paired *t* test

    D. Student's *t* test

    E. Logistic regression analysis

13.14. Suppose that we are interested in studying the association between being exposed to second-hand smoke and having a low birth-weight infant. To study this association, we identify 50 women who have recently delivered a singleton infant and who were exposed to second-hand smoke during their pregnancy and 50 women who have recently delivered a singleton infant and who were not exposed to second-hand smoke during their pregnancy. For each of these women we determine the birth-weight of their infant. Now, suppose we define a low birth weight as being less than 1,500 grams. Which of the following is the common name of the statistical procedure that would be best to use to compare the odds of having a low birth weight infant between these two groups of women?

    A. Fisher's exact test

    B. McNemar's test

    C. Paired *t* test

    D. Student's *t* test

    E. Logistic regression analysis

13.15. Suppose that we are interested in studying the association between being exposed to second-hand smoke and having a low birth-weight infant. To study this association, we identify 50 women who have recently delivered a singleton infant and who were exposed to second-hand smoke during their pregnancy and 50 women who have recently delivered a singleton infant and who were not exposed to second-hand smoke during their pregnancy. For each of these women we determine the birth-weight of their infant. Now, suppose we define a low birth weight as being less than 1,500 grams. Which of the following is the common name of the statistical procedure that would be best to use to compare the odds of having a low birth weight infant between these two groups of women while controlling for the confounding effect of maternal age?

    A. Fisher's exact test

    B. McNemar's test

    C. Paired *t* test

    D. Student's *t* test

    E. Logistic regression analysis

APPENDIX A

FLOWCHARTS

Chapters 4 through 12 in the textbook are structured to reflect the thinking process of statisticians when choosing a statistical method to analyze a particular set of data. At the beginning of each of those chapters, the methods discussed in that chapter appear in a flowchart that summarizes statisticians' thinking process. In this appendix, we have brought those flowcharts together so they are easier to use. As explained in the introduction to Part Two of the textbook, you should start by using the master flowchart (designated as Flowchart 1 in the text) that appears below. Following the steps in this flowchart will lead to the chapter of the text that discusses the types of statistical methods that might be used to analyze a particular set of data. The flowcharts following the master flowchart in this appendix are labeled according to the textbook chapter in which they are discussed. Examining these flowcharts will reveal the most commonly used statistical methods to analyze your data.

In each of the subsequent flowcharts, the estimate that is most often used to describe the dependent variable is in italics, the common name of the statistical test is enclosed in a box, the standard distribution (or approach) that is used to test hypotheses and/or calculate confidence intervals is in bold.

Workbook to Accompany Introduction to Biostatistical Applications in Health Research with Microsoft® Office Excel®, First Edition. Robert P. Hirsch.
© 2016 John Wiley & Sons, Inc. Published 2016 by John Wiley & Sons, Inc.

MASTER FLOWCHART

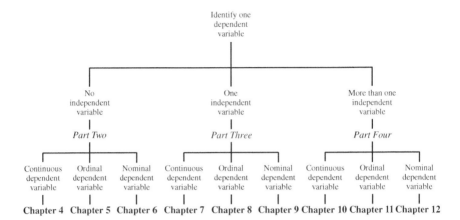

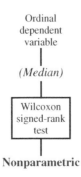

Student's t

CHAPTER 4. Univariable analysis of a continuous dependent variable.

Ordinal
dependent
variable

(Median)

Wilcoxon
signed-rank
test

Nonparametric

CHAPTER 5. Univariable analysis of an ordinal dependent variable.

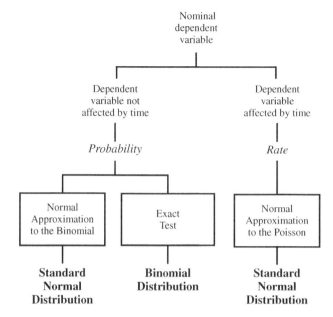

CHAPTER 6. Univariable analysis of a nominal dependent variable.

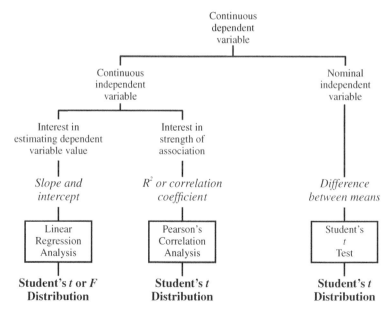

CHAPTER 7. Bivariable analysis of a continuous dependent variable.

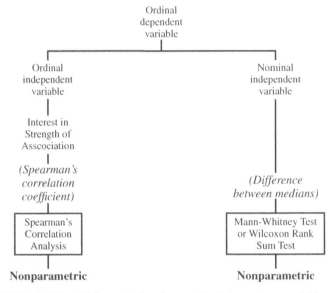

CHAPTER 8. Bivariable analysis of an ordinal dependent variable.

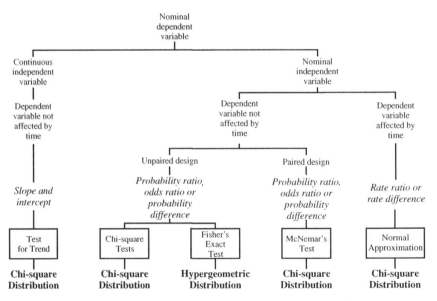

CHAPTER 9. Bivariable analysis of a nominal dependent variable.

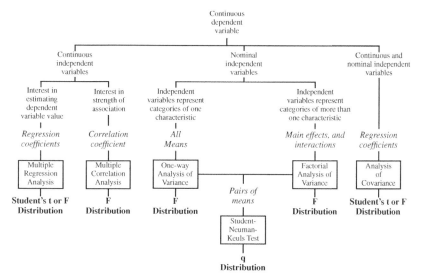

CHAPTER 10. Multivariable analysis of a continuous dependent variable.

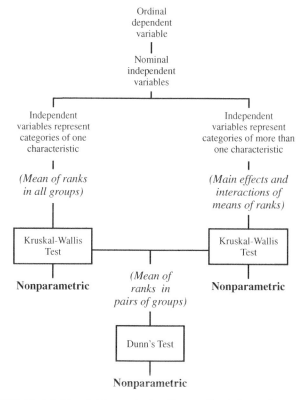

CHAPTER 11. Multivariable analysis of an ordinal dependent variable.

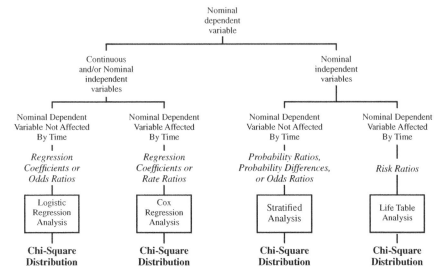

CHAPTER 12. Multivariable analysis of a nominal dependent variable.

APPENDIX B

STATISTICAL TABLES

Workbook to Accompany Introduction to Biostatistical Applications in Health Research with Microsoft® Office Excel®, First Edition. Robert P. Hirsch.
© 2016 John Wiley & Sons, Inc. Published 2016 by John Wiley & Sons, Inc.

Table B.1   Area in one tail of the standard normal distribution[*]

z	0	1	2	3	4	5	6	7	8	9
0.0	0.5000	0.4960	0.4920	0.4880	0.4840	0.4801	0.4761	0.4721	0.4681	0.4641
0.1	0.4602	0.4562	0.4522	0.4483	0.4443	0.4404	0.4364	0.4325	0.4286	0.4247
0.2	0.4207	0.4168	0.4129	0.4090	0.4052	0.4013	0.3974	0.3936	0.3897	0.3859
0.3	0.3821	0.3783	0.3745	0.3707	0.3669	0.3632	0.3594	0.3557	0.3520	0.3483
0.4	0.3446	0.3409	0.3372	0.3336	0.3300	0.3264	0.3228	0.3192	0.3156	0.3121
0.5	0.3085	0.3050	0.3015	0.2981	0.2946	0.2912	0.2877	0.2843	0.2810	0.2776
0.6	0.2743	0.2709	0.2676	0.2643	0.2611	0.2578	0.2546	0.2514	0.2483	0.2451
0.7	0.2420	0.2389	0.2358	0.2327	0.2297	0.2266	0.2236	0.2207	0.2177	0.2148
0.8	0.2119	0.2090	0.2061	0.2033	0.2005	0.1977	0.1949	0.1922	0.1894	0.1867
0.9	0.1841	0.1814	0.1788	0.1762	0.1736	0.1711	0.1685	0.1660	0.1635	0.1611
1.0	0.1587	0.1562	0.1539	0.1515	0.1492	0.1469	0.1446	0.1423	0.1401	0.1379
1.1	0.1357	0.1335	0.1314	0.1292	0.1271	0.1251	0.1230	0.1210	0.1190	0.1170
1.2	0.1151	0.1131	0.1112	0.1093	0.1075	0.1056	0.1038	0.1020	0.1003	0.0985
1.3	0.0968	0.0951	0.0934	0.0918	0.0901	0.0885	0.0869	0.0853	0.0838	0.0823
1.4	0.0808	0.0793	0.0778	0.0764	0.0749	0.0735	0.0721	0.0708	0.0694	0.0681
1.5	0.0668	0.0655	0.0643	0.0630	0.0618	0.0606	0.0594	0.0582	0.0571	0.0559
1.6	0.0548	0.0537	0.0526	0.0516	0.0505	0.0495	0.0485	0.0475	0.0465	0.0455
1.7	0.0446	0.0436	0.0427	0.0418	0.0409	0.0401	0.0392	0.0384	0.0375	0.0367
1.8	0.0359	0.0351	0.0344	0.0336	0.0329	0.0322	0.0314	0.0307	0.0301	0.0294
1.9	0.0287	0.0281	0.0274	0.0268	0.0262	0.0256	0.0250	0.0244	0.0239	0.0233
2.0	0.0228	0.0222	0.0217	0.0212	0.0207	0.0202	0.0197	0.0192	0.0188	0.0183
2.1	0.0179	0.0174	0.0170	0.0166	0.0162	0.0158	0.0154	0.0150	0.0146	0.0143
2.2	0.0139	0.0136	0.0132	0.0129	0.0125	0.0122	0.0119	0.0116	0.0113	0.0110
2.3	0.0107	0.0104	0.0102	0.0099	0.0096	0.0094	0.0091	0.0089	0.0087	0.0084
2.4	0.0082	0.0080	0.0078	0.0075	0.0073	0.0071	0.0069	0.0068	0.0066	0.0064
2.5	0.0062	0.0060	0.0059	0.0057	0.0055	0.0054	0.0052	0.0051	0.0049	0.0048
2.6	0.0047	0.0045	0.0044	0.0043	0.0041	0.0040	0.0039	0.0038	0.0037	0.0036
2.7	0.0035	0.0034	0.0033	0.0032	0.0031	0.0030	0.0029	0.0028	0.0027	0.0026
2.8	0.0026	0.0025	0.0024	0.0023	0.0023	0.0022	0.0021	0.0021	0.0020	0.0019
2.9	0.0019	0.0018	0.0018	0.0017	0.0016	0.0016	0.0015	0.0015	0.0014	0.0014
3.0	0.0013	0.0013	0.0013	0.0012	0.0012	0.0011	0.0011	0.0011	0.0010	0.0010
3.1	0.0010	0.0009	0.0009	0.0009	0.0008	0.0008	0.0008	0.0008	0.0007	0.0007
3.2	0.0007	0.0007	0.0006	0.0006	0.0006	0.0006	0.0006	0.0005	0.0005	0.0005
3.3	0.0005	0.0005	0.0005	0.0004	0.0004	0.0004	0.0004	0.0004	0.0004	0.0003
3.4	0.0003	0.0003	0.0003	0.0003	0.0003	0.0003	0.0003	0.0003	0.0003	0.0002
3.5	0.0002	0.0002	0.0002	0.0002	0.0002	0.0002	0.0002	0.0002	0.0002	0.0002
3.6	0.0002	0.0002	0.0001	0.0001	0.0001	0.0001	0.0001	0.0001	0.0001	0.0001
3.7	0.0001	0.0001	0.0001	0.0001	0.0001	0.0001	0.0001	0.0001	0.0001	0.0001
3.8	0.0001	0.0001	0.0001	0.0001	0.0001	0.0001	0.0001	0.0001	0.0001	0.0001

[*]To determine the area in one tail of the standard normal distribution, calculate a standard normal deviate (z) to two decimal places. Find the first two digits of that deviate (units and tenths) in the left-hand column. Find the third digit (hundredths) in the top row. The corresponding area is at the intersection of that column and that row.

Table B.2   Critical values of Student's t distribution*

$\alpha(2)$	0.50	0.20	0.10	0.05	0.02	0.01	0.005	0.002	0.001
$\alpha(1)$	0.25	0.10	0.05	0.025	0.01	0.005	0.0025	0.001	0.0005
df									
1	1.000	3.078	6.314	12.71	31.82	63.66	127.3	318.3	636.6
2	0.816	1.886	2.920	4.303	6.965	9.925	14.09	22.33	31.60
3	0.765	1.638	2.353	3.182	4.541	5.841	7.453	10.22	12.92
4	0.741	1.533	2.132	2.776	3.747	4.604	5.598	7.173	8.610
5	0.727	1.476	2.015	2.571	3.365	4.032	4.773	5.893	6.869
6	0.718	1.440	1.943	2.447	3.143	3.707	4.317	5.208	5.959
7	0.711	1.415	1.895	2.365	2.998	3.499	4.029	4.785	5.408
8	0.706	1.397	1.860	2.306	2.896	3.355	3.833	4.501	5.041
9	0.703	1.383	1.833	2.262	2.821	3.250	3.690	4.297	4.781
10	0.700	1.372	1.812	2.228	2.764	3.169	3.581	4.144	4.587
11	0.697	1.363	1.796	2.201	2.718	3.106	3.497	4.025	4.437
12	0.695	1.356	1.782	2.179	2.681	3.055	3.428	3.930	4.318
13	0.694	1.350	1.771	2.160	2.650	3.012	3.372	3.852	4.221
14	0.692	1.345	1.761	2.145	2.624	2.977	3.326	3.787	4.140
15	0.691	1.341	1.753	2.131	2.602	2.947	3.286	3.733	4.073
16	0.690	1.337	1.746	2.120	2.583	2.921	3.252	3.686	4.015
17	0.689	1.333	1.740	2.110	2.567	2.898	3.222	3.646	3.965
18	0.688	1.330	1.734	2.101	2.552	2.878	3.197	3.610	3.922
19	0.688	1.328	1.729	2.093	2.539	2.861	3.174	3.579	3.883
20	0.687	1.325	1.725	2.086	2.528	2.845	3.153	3.552	3.850
22	0.686	1.321	1.717	2.074	2.508	2.819	3.119	3.505	3.792
24	0.685	1.318	1.711	2.064	2.492	2.797	3.091	3.467	3.745
26	0.684	1.315	1.706	2.056	2.479	2.779	3.067	3.435	3.707
28	0.683	1.313	1.701	2.048	2.467	2.763	3.047	3.408	3.674
30	0.683	1.310	1.697	2.042	2.457	2.750	3.030	3.385	3.646
32	0.682	1.309	1.694	2.037	2.449	2.738	3.015	3.365	3.622
34	0.682	1.307	1.691	2.032	2.441	2.728	3.002	3.348	3.601
36	0.681	1.306	1.688	2.028	2.434	2.719	2.990	3.333	3.582
38	0.681	1.304	1.686	2.024	2.429	2.712	2.980	3.319	3.566
40	0.681	1.303	1.684	2.021	2.423	2.704	2.971	3.307	3.551
45	0.680	1.301	1.679	2.014	2.412	2.690	2.952	3.281	3.520
50	0.679	1.299	1.676	2.009	2.403	2.678	2.937	3.261	3.496
55	0.679	1.297	1.674	2.004	2.396	2.668	2.925	3.245	3.477
60	0.679	1.296	1.671	2.000	2.390	2.660	2.915	3.232	3.460
65	0.678	1.295	1.669	1.997	2.385	2.654	2.906	3.221	3.447
70	0.678	1.294	1.667	1.994	2.381	2.648	2.899	3.211	3.435
75	0.678	1.293	1.665	1.992	2.377	2.643	2.893	3.203	3.425
80	0.678	1.292	1.664	1.990	2.374	2.639	2.887	3.195	3.416
85	0.677	1.291	1.663	1.988	2.371	2.635	2.882	3.189	3.409
90	0.677	1.291	1.662	1.987	2.368	2.632	2.878	3.183	3.402
100	0.677	1.290	1.660	1.984	2.364	2.626	2.871	3.174	3.390
150	0.676	1.287	1.655	1.976	2.351	2.609	2.849	3.145	3.357
200	0.676	1.286	1.653	1.972	2.345	2.601	2.839	3.131	3.340
500	0.675	1.283	1.648	1.965	2.334	2.586	2.820	3.107	3.310
∞	0.674	1.282	1.645	1.960	2.326	2.576	2.807	3.090	3.290

*To locate Student's t value, find the degrees of freedom in the leftmost column and the appropriate α at the top of the table ($\alpha(2)$ indicates a two-tailed value and $\alpha(1)$ indicates a one-tailed value). The number in the body of the table where this row and column intersect is Student's t value from a distribution with that number of degrees of freedom and that corresponds to an area equal to α.

Table B.3 Critical values of Wilcoxon's T statistic*

$\alpha(2)$	0.50	0.20	0.10	0.05	0.02	0.01	0.005	0.001
$\alpha(1)$	0.25	0.10	0.05	0.025	0.01	0.005	0.0025	0.0005
n								
4	2	0						
5	4	2	0					
6	6	3	2	0				
7	9	5	3	2	0			
8	12	8	5	3	1	0		
9	16	10	8	5	3	1	0	
10	20	14	10	8	5	3	1	
11	24	17	13	10	7	5	3	0
12	29	21	17	13	9	7	5	1
13	35	26	21	17	12	9	7	2
14	40	31	25	21	15	12	9	4
15	47	36	30	25	19	15	12	6
16	54	42	35	29	23	19	15	8
17	61	48	41	34	27	23	19	11
18	69	55	47	40	32	27	23	14
19	77	62	53	46	37	32	27	18
20	86	69	60	52	43	37	32	21
21	95	77	67	58	49	42	37	25
22	104	86	75	65	55	48	42	30
23	114	94	83	73	62	54	48	35
24	125	104	91	81	69	61	54	40
25	136	113	100	89	76	68	60	45
26	148	124	110	98	84	75	67	51
27	160	134	119	107	92	83	74	57
28	172	145	130	116	101	91	82	64
29	185	157	140	126	110	100	90	71
30	198	169	151	137	120	109	98	78
32	226	194	175	159	140	128	116	94
34	257	221	200	182	162	148	136	111
36	289	250	227	208	185	171	157	130
38	323	281	256	235	211	194	180	150
40	358	313	286	264	238	220	204	172
42	396	348	319	294	266	247	230	195
44	436	384	353	327	296	276	258	220
46	477	422	389	361	328	307	287	246
48	521	462	426	396	362	339	318	274
50	566	503	466	434	397	373	350	304
55	688	615	573	536	493	465	438	385
60	822	739	690	648	600	567	537	476
65	968	875	820	772	718	681	647	577
70	1126	1022	960	907	846	805	767	689
75	1296	1181	1112	1053	986	940	898	811
80	1478	1351	1276	1211	1136	1086	1039	943
85	1672	1533	1451	1380	1298	1242	1191	1086
90	1878	1727	1638	1560	1471	1410	1355	1240
95	2097	1933	1836	1752	1655	1589	1529	1404
100	2327	2151	2045	1955	1850	1779	1714	1578

*To locate Wilcoxon's T value, find the sample's size in the leftmost column and the appropriate α at the top of the table ($\alpha(2)$ indicates a two-tailed value and $\alpha(1)$ indicates a one-tailed value). A calculated T value is statistically significant (i.e., the null hypothesis can be rejected) if it is equal to or less than the value in the table.

Table B.4 Critical values of the F distribution*

	Numerator df = 1								
α(↓)	0.25	0.10	0.05	0.025	0.01	0.005	0.0025	0.001	0.0005
Denom df									
1	5.83	39.9	161.	648.	4050.	16200.	64800.	$4 \cdot 10^5$	$2 \cdot 10^6$
2	2.57	8.53	18.5	38.5	98.5	199.	399.	999.0	2000.
3	2.02	5.54	10.1	17.4	34.1	55.6	89.6	167.	267.
4	1.81	4.54	7.71	12.2	21.2	31.3	45.7	74.1	106.
5	1.69	4.06	6.61	10.0	16.3	22.8	31.4	47.2	63.6
6	1.62	3.78	5.99	8.81	13.7	18.6	24.8	35.5	46.1
7	1.57	3.59	5.59	8.07	12.2	16.2	21.1	29.2	37.0
8	1.54	3.46	5.32	7.57	11.3	14.7	18.8	25.4	31.6
9	1.51	3.36	5.12	7.21	10.6	13.6	17.2	22.9	28.0
10	1.49	3.29	4.96	6.94	10.0	12.8	16.0	21.0	25.5
11	1.47	3.23	4.84	6.72	9.65	12.2	15.2	19.7	23.7
12	1.46	3.18	4.75	6.55	9.33	11.8	14.5	18.6	22.2
13	1.45	3.14	4.67	6.41	9.07	11.4	13.9	17.8	21.1
14	1.44	3.10	4.60	6.30	8.86	11.1	13.5	17.1	20.2
15	1.43	3.07	4.54	6.20	8.68	10.8	13.1	16.6	19.5
16	1.42	3.05	4.49	6.12	8.53	10.6	12.8	16.1	18.9
17	1.42	3.03	4.45	6.04	8.40	10.4	12.6	15.7	18.4
18	1.41	3.01	4.41	5.98	8.29	10.2	12.3	15.4	17.9
19	1.41	2.99	4.38	5.92	8.18	10.1	12.1	15.1	17.5
20	1.40	2.97	4.35	5.87	8.10	9.94	11.9	14.8	17.2
21	1.40	2.96	4.32	5.83	8.02	9.83	11.8	14.6	16.9
22	1.40	2.95	4.30	5.79	7.95	9.73	11.6	14.4	16.6
23	1.39	2.94	4.28	5.75	7.88	9.63	11.5	14.2	16.4
24	1.39	2.93	4.26	5.72	7.82	9.55	11.4	14.0	16.2
25	1.39	2.92	4.24	5.69	7.77	9.48	11.3	13.9	16.0
26	1.38	2.91	4.23	5.66	7.72	9.41	11.2	13.7	15.8
27	1.38	2.90	4.21	5.63	7.68	9.34	11.1	13.6	15.6
28	1.38	2.89	4.20	5.61	7.64	9.28	11.0	13.5	15.5
29	1.38	2.89	4.18	5.59	7.60	9.23	11.0	13.4	15.3
30	1.38	2.88	4.17	5.57	7.56	9.18	10.9	13.3	15.2
35	1.37	2.85	4.12	5.48	7.42	8.98	10.6	12.9	14.7
40	1.36	2.84	4.08	5.42	7.31	8.83	10.4	12.6	14.4
45	1.36	2.82	4.06	5.38	7.23	8.71	10.3	12.4	14.1
50	1.35	2.81	4.03	5.34	7.17	8.63	10.1	12.2	13.9
60	1.35	2.79	4.00	5.29	7.08	8.49	9.96	12.0	13.5
70	1.35	2.78	3.98	5.25	7.01	8.40	9.84	11.8	13.3
80	1.34	2.77	3.96	5.22	6.96	8.33	9.75	11.7	13.2
90	1.34	2.76	3.95	5.20	6.93	8.28	9.68	11.6	13.0
100	1.34	2.76	3.94	5.18	6.90	8.24	9.62	11.5	12.9
200	1.33	2.73	3.89	5.10	6.76	8.06	9.38	11.2	12.5
500	1.33	2.72	3.86	5.05	6.69	7.95	9.23	11.0	12.3
∞	1.32	2.71	3.84	5.02	6.64	7.88	9.14	10.8	12.1

*To locate an F value, first find the table that is headed by the degrees of freedom in the numerator of your F ratio. Then, find the degrees of freedom in the denominator of your F ratio in the leftmost column. Finally, find the appropriate α at the top of the table. The number in the body of the table where this row and column intersect is the F statistic from a distribution with those numerator and denominator degrees of freedom and that corresponds to an area of α in one tail of the F distribution.

Table B.4 *Continued*

				Numerator df = 2					
$\alpha(1)$	0.25	0.10	0.05	0.025	0.01	0.005	0.0025	0.001	0.0005
Denom df									
1	7.50	49.5	200.	800.	5000.	20000.	80000.	$5 \cdot 10^5$	$2 \cdot 10^6$
2	3.00	9.00	19.0	39.0	99.0	199.	399.	999.	2000.
3	2.28	5.46	9.55	16.0	30.8	49.8	79.0	149.	237.
4	2.00	4.32	6.94	10.6	18.0	26.3	38.0	61.2	87.4
5	1.85	3.78	5.79	8.43	13.3	18.3	25.0	37.1	49.8
6	1.76	3.46	5.14	7.26	10.9	14.5	19.1	27.0	34.8
7	1.70	3.26	4.74	6.54	9.55	12.4	15.9	21.7	27.2
8	1.66	3.11	4.46	6.06	8.65	11.0	13.9	18.5	22.7
9	1.62	3.01	4.26	5.71	8.02	10.1	12.5	16.4	19.9
10	1.60	2.92	4.10	5.46	7.56	9.43	11.6	14.9	17.9
11	1.58	2.86	3.98	5.26	7.21	8.91	10.8	13.8	16.4
12	1.56	2.81	3.89	5.10	6.93	8.51	10.3	13.0	15.3
13	1.55	2.76	3.81	4.97	6.70	8.19	9.84	12.3	14.4
14	1.53	2.73	3.74	4.86	6.51	7.92	9.47	11.8	13.7
15	1.52	2.70	3.68	4.77	6.36	7.70	9.17	11.3	13.2
16	1.51	2.67	3.63	4.69	6.23	7.51	8.92	11.0	12.7
17	1.51	2.64	3.59	4.62	6.11	7.35	8.70	10.7	12.3
18	1.50	2.62	3.55	4.56	6.01	7.21	8.51	10.4	11.9
19	1.49	2.61	3.52	4.51	5.93	7.09	8.35	10.2	11.6
20	1.49	2.59	3.49	4.46	5.85	6.99	8.21	9.95	11.4
21	1.48	2.57	3.47	4.42	5.78	6.89	8.08	9.77	11.2
22	1.48	2.56	3.44	4.38	5.72	6.81	7.96	9.61	11.0
23	1.47	2.55	3.42	4.35	5.66	6.73	7.86	9.47	10.8
24	1.47	2.54	3.40	4.32	5.61	6.66	7.77	9.34	10.6
25	1.47	2.53	3.39	4.29	5.57	6.60	7.69	9.22	10.5
26	1.46	2.52	3.37	4.27	5.53	6.54	7.61	9.12	10.3
27	1.46	2.51	3.35	4.24	5.49	6.49	7.54	9.02	10.2
28	1.46	2.50	3.34	4.22	5.45	6.44	7.48	8.93	10.1
29	1.45	2.50	3.33	4.20	5.42	6.40	7.42	8.85	9.99
30	1.45	2.49	3.32	4.18	5.39	6.35	7.36	8.77	9.90
35	1.44	2.46	3.27	4.11	5.27	6.19	7.14	8.47	9.52
40	1.44	2.44	3.23	4.05	5.18	6.07	6.99	8.25	9.25
45	1.43	2.42	3.20	4.01	5.11	5.97	6.86	8.09	9.04
50	1.43	2.41	3.18	3.97	5.06	5.90	6.77	7.96	8.88
60	1.42	2.39	3.15	3.93	4.98	5.79	6.63	7.77	8.65
70	1.41	2.38	3.13	3.89	4.92	5.72	6.53	7.64	8.49
80	1.41	2.37	3.11	3.86	4.88	5.67	6.46	7.54	8.37
90	1.41	2.36	3.10	3.84	4.85	5.62	6.41	7.47	8.28
100	1.41	2.36	3.09	3.83	4.82	5.59	6.37	7.41	8.21
200	1.40	2.33	3.04	3.76	4.71	5.44	6.17	7.15	7.90
500	1.39	2.31	3.01	3.72	4.65	5.35	6.06	7.00	7.72
∞	1.39	2.30	3.00	3.69	4.61	5.30	5.99	6.91	7.60

Table B.4 *Continued*

	Numerator df = 3								
$\alpha(1)$	0.25	0.10	0.05	0.025	0.01	0.005	0.0025	0.001	0.0005
Denom df									
1	8.20	53.6	216.	864.	5400.	21600.	86500.	$5 \cdot 10^5$	$2 \cdot 10^6$
2	3.15	9.16	19.2	39.2	99.2	199.	399.	999.	2000.
3	2.36	5.39	9.28	15.4	29.5	47.5	76.1	141.	225.
4	2.05	4.19	6.59	9.98	16.7	24.3	35.0	56.2	80.1
5	1.88	3.62	5.41	7.76	12.1	16.5	22.4	33.2	44.4
6	1.78	3.29	4.76	6.60	9.78	12.9	16.9	23.7	30.5
7	1.72	3.07	4.35	5.89	8.45	10.9	13.8	18.8	23.5
8	1.67	2.92	4.07	5.42	7.59	9.60	12.0	15.8	19.4
9	1.63	2.81	3.86	5.08	6.99	8.72	10.7	13.9	16.8
10	1.60	2.73	3.71	4.83	6.55	8.08	9.83	12.6	15.0
11	1.58	2.66	3.59	4.63	6.22	7.60	9.17	11.6	13.7
12	1.56	2.61	3.49	4.47	5.95	7.23	8.65	10.8	12.7
13	1.55	2.56	3.41	4.35	5.74	6.93	8.24	10.2	11.9
14	1.53	2.52	3.34	4.24	5.56	6.68	7.91	9.73	11.3
15	1.52	2.49	3.29	4.15	5.42	6.48	7.63	9.34	10.8
16	1.51	2.46	3.24	4.08	5.29	6.30	7.40	9.01	10.3
17	1.50	2.44	3.20	4.01	5.19	6.16	7.21	8.73	9.99
18	1.49	2.42	3.16	3.95	5.09	6.03	7.04	8.49	9.69
19	1.49	2.40	3.13	3.90	5.01	5.92	6.89	8.28	9.42
20	1.48	2.38	3.10	3.86	4.94	5.82	6.76	8.10	9.20
21	1.48	2.36	3.07	3.82	4.87	5.73	6.64	7.94	8.99
22	1.47	2.35	3.05	3.78	4.82	5.65	6.54	7.80	8.82
23	1.47	2.34	3.03	3.75	4.76	5.58	6.45	7.67	8.66
24	1.46	2.33	3.01	3.72	4.72	5.52	6.36	7.55	8.51
25	1.46	2.32	2.99	3.69	4.68	5.46	6.29	7.45	8.39
26	1.45	2.31	2.98	3.67	4.64	5.41	6.22	7.36	8.27
27	1.45	2.30	2.96	3.65	4.60	5.36	6.16	7.27	8.16
28	1.45	2.29	2.95	3.63	4.57	5.32	6.10	7.19	8.07
29	1.45	2.28	2.93	3.61	4.54	5.28	6.05	7.12	7.98
30	1.44	2.28	2.92	3.59	4.51	5.24	6.00	7.05	7.89
35	1.43	2.25	2.87	3.52	4.40	5.09	5.80	6.79	7.56
40	1.42	2.23	2.84	3.46	4.31	4.98	5.66	6.59	7.33
45	1.42	2.21	2.81	3.42	4.25	4.89	5.55	6.45	7.15
50	1.41	2.20	2.79	3.39	4.20	4.83	5.47	6.34	7.01
60	1.41	2.18	2.76	3.34	4.13	4.73	5.34	6.17	6.81
70	1.40	2.16	2.74	3.31	4.07	4.66	5.26	6.06	6.67
80	1.40	2.15	2.72	3.28	4.04	4.61	5.19	5.97	6.57
90	1.39	2.15	2.71	3.26	4.01	4.57	5.14	5.91	6.49
100	1.39	2.14	2.70	3.25	3.98	4.54	5.11	5.86	6.43
200	1.38	2.11	2.65	3.18	3.88	4.41	4.94	5.63	6.16
500	1.37	2.09	2.62	3.14	3.82	4.33	4.84	5.51	6.01
∞	1.37	2.08	2.62	3.12	3.78	4.28	4.77	5.42	5.91

Table B.4 *Continued*

				Numerator df = 4					
$\alpha(1)$	0.25	0.10	0.05	0.025	0.01	0.005	0.0025	0.001	0.0005
Denom df									
1	8.58	55.8	225.	900.	5620.	22500.	90000.	$6 \cdot 10^5$	$2 \cdot 10^6$
2	3.23	9.24	19.2	39.2	99.2	199.	399.	999.	2000.
3	2.39	5.34	9.12	15.1	28.7	46.2	73.9	137.	218.
4	2.06	4.11	6.39	9.60	16.0	23.2	33.3	53.4	76.1
5	1.89	3.52	5.19	7.39	11.4	15.6	21.0	31.1	41.5
6	1.79	3.18	4.53	6.23	9.15	12.0	15.7	21.9	28.1
7	1.72	2.96	4.12	5.52	7.85	10.1	12.7	17.2	21.4
8	1.66	2.81	3.84	5.05	7.01	8.81	10.9	14.4	17.6
9	1.63	2.69	3.63	4.72	6.42	7.96	9.74	12.6	15.1
10	1.59	2.61	3.48	4.47	5.99	7.34	8.89	11.3	13.4
11	1.57	2.54	3.36	4.28	5.67	6.88	8.25	10.3	12.2
12	1.55	2.48	3.26	4.12	5.41	6.52	7.76	9.63	11.2
13	1.53	2.43	3.18	4.00	5.21	6.23	7.37	9.07	10.5
14	1.52	2.39	3.11	3.89	5.04	6.00	7.06	8.62	9.95
15	1.51	2.36	3.06	3.80	4.89	5.80	6.80	8.25	9.48
16	1.50	2.33	3.01	3.73	4.77	5.64	6.58	7.94	9.08
17	1.49	2.31	2.96	3.66	4.67	5.50	6.39	7.68	8.75
18	1.48	2.29	2.93	3.61	4.58	5.37	6.23	7.46	8.47
19	1.47	2.27	2.90	3.56	4.50	5.27	6.09	7.27	8.23
20	1.47	2.25	2.87	3.51	4.43	5.17	5.97	7.10	8.02
21	1.46	2.23	2.84	3.48	4.37	5.09	5.86	6.95	7.83
22	1.45	2.22	2.82	3.44	4.31	5.02	5.76	6.81	7.67
23	1.45	2.21	2.80	3.41	4.26	4.95	5.67	6.70	7.52
24	1.44	2.19	2.78	3.38	4.22	4.89	5.60	6.59	7.39
25	1.44	2.18	2.76	3.35	4.18	4.84	5.53	6.49	7.27
26	1.44	2.17	2.74	3.33	4.14	4.79	5.46	6.41	7.16
27	1.43	2.17	2.73	3.31	4.11	4.74	5.40	6.33	7.06
28	1.43	2.16	2.71	3.29	4.07	4.70	5.35	6.25	6.97
29	1.43	2.15	2.70	3.27	4.04	4.66	5.30	6.19	6.89
30	1.42	2.14	2.69	3.25	4.02	4.62	5.25	6.12	6.82
35	1.41	2.11	2.64	3.18	3.91	4.48	5.07	5.88	6.51
40	1.40	2.09	2.61	3.13	3.83	4.37	4.93	5.70	6.30
45	1.40	2.07	2.58	3.09	3.77	4.29	4.83	5.56	6.13
50	1.39	2.06	2.56	3.05	3.72	4.23	4.75	5.46	6.01
60	1.38	2.04	2.53	3.01	3.65	4.14	4.64	5.31	5.82
70	1.38	2.03	2.50	2.97	3.60	4.08	4.56	5.20	5.70
80	1.38	2.02	2.49	2.95	3.56	4.03	4.50	5.12	5.60
90	1.37	2.01	2.47	2.93	3.53	3.99	4.45	5.06	5.53
100	1.37	2.00	2.46	2.92	3.51	3.96	4.42	5.02	5.48
200	1.36	1.97	2.42	2.85	3.41	3.84	4.26	4.81	5.23
500	1.35	1.96	2.39	2.81	3.36	3.76	4.17	4.69	5.09
∞	1.35	1.94	2.37	2.79	3.32	3.72	4.11	4.62	5.00

Table B.4 *Continued*

				Numerator df = 5					
$\alpha(1)$	0.25	0.10	0.05	0.025	0.01	0.005	0.0025	0.001	0.0005
Denom df									
1	8.82	57.2	230.	922.	5760.	23100.	92200.	$6 \cdot 10^5$	$2 \cdot 10^6$
2	3.28	9.29	19.3	39.3	99.3	199.	399.	999.	2000.
3	2.41	5.31	9.01	14.9	28.2	45.4	72.6	135.	214.
4	2.07	4.05	6.26	9.36	15.5	22.5	32.3	51.7	73.6
5	1.89	3.45	5.05	7.15	11.0	14.9	20.2	29.8	39.7
6	1.79	3.11	4.39	5.99	8.75	11.5	14.9	20.8	26.6
7	1.71	2.88	3.97	5.29	7.46	9.52	12.0	16.2	20.2
8	1.66	2.73	3.69	4.82	6.63	8.30	10.3	13.5	16.4
9	1.62	2.61	3.48	4.48	6.06	7.47	9.12	11.7	14.1
10	1.59	2.52	3.33	4.24	5.64	6.87	8.29	10.5	12.4
11	1.56	2.45	3.20	4.04	5.32	6.42	7.67	9.58	11.2
12	1.54	2.39	3.11	3.89	5.06	6.07	7.20	8.89	10.4
13	1.52	2.35	3.03	3.77	4.86	5.79	6.82	8.35	9.66
14	1.51	2.31	2.96	3.66	4.69	5.56	6.51	7.92	9.11
15	1.49	2.27	2.90	3.58	4.56	5.37	6.26	7.57	8.66
16	1.48	2.24	2.85	3.50	4.44	5.21	6.05	7.27	8.29
17	1.47	2.22	2.81	3.44	4.34	5.07	5.87	7.02	7.98
18	1.46	2.20	2.77	3.38	4.25	4.96	5.72	6.81	7.71
19	1.46	2.18	2.74	3.33	4.17	4.85	5.58	6.62	7.48
20	1.45	2.16	2.71	3.29	4.10	4.76	5.46	6.46	7.27
21	1.44	2.14	2.68	3.25	4.04	4.68	5.36	6.32	7.10
22	1.44	2.13	2.66	3.22	3.99	4.61	5.26	6.19	6.94
23	1.43	2.11	2.64	3.18	3.94	4.54	5.18	6.08	6.80
24	1.43	2.10	2.62	3.15	3.90	4.49	5.11	5.98	6.68
25	1.42	2.09	2.60	3.13	3.85	4.43	5.04	5.89	6.56
26	1.42	2.08	2.59	3.10	3.82	4.38	4.98	5.80	6.46
27	1.42	2.07	2.57	3.08	3.78	4.34	4.92	5.73	7.37
28	1.41	2.06	2.56	3.06	3.75	4.30	4.87	5.66	6.28
29	1.41	2.06	2.55	3.04	3.73	4.26	4.82	5.59	6.21
30	1.41	2.05	2.53	3.03	3.70	4.23	4.78	5.53	6.13
35	1.40	2.02	2.49	2.96	3.59	4.09	4.60	5.30	5.85
40	1.39	2.00	2.45	2.90	3.51	3.99	4.47	5.13	5.64
45	1.38	1.98	2.42	2.86	3.45	3.91	4.37	5.00	5.49
50	1.37	1.97	2.40	2.83	3.41	3.85	4.30	4.90	5.37
60	1.37	1.95	2.37	2.79	3.34	3.76	4.19	4.76	5.20
70	1.36	1.93	2.35	2.75	3.29	3.70	4.11	4.66	5.08
80	1.36	1.92	2.33	2.73	3.26	3.65	4.05	4.58	4.99
90	1.35	1.91	2.32	2.71	3.23	3.62	4.01	4.53	4.92
100	1.35	1.91	2.31	2.70	3.21	3.59	3.97	4.48	4.87
200	1.34	1.88	2.26	2.63	3.11	3.47	3.82	4.29	4.64
500	1.33	1.86	2.23	2.59	3.05	3.40	3.73	4.18	4.51
∞	1.33	1.85	2.22	2.57	3.02	3.35	3.68	4.10	4.42

Table B.4 *Continued*

α(!)	0.25	0.10	0.05	0.025	0.01	0.005	0.0025	0.001	0.0005
	Numerator df = 6								
Denom df									
1	8.98	58.2	234.	937.	5860.	23400.	93700.	$6 \cdot 10^5$	$2 \cdot 10^6$
2	3.31	9.33	19.3	39.3	99.3	199.	399.	999.	2000.
3	2.42	5.28	8.94	14.7	27.9	44.8	71.7	133.	211.9
4	2.08	4.01	6.16	9.20	15.2	22.0	31.5	50.5	71.9
5	1.89	3.40	4.95	6.98	10.7	14.5	19.6	28.8	38.5
6	1.78	3.05	4.28	5.82	8.47	11.1	14.4	20.0	25.6
7	1.71	2.83	3.87	5.12	7.19	9.16	11.5	15.5	19.3
8	1.65	2.67	3.58	4.65	6.37	7.95	9.83	12.9	15.7
9	1.61	2.55	3.37	4.32	5.80	7.13	8.68	11.1	13.3
10	1.58	2.46	3.22	4.07	5.39	6.54	7.87	9.93	11.7
11	1.55	2.39	3.09	3.88	5.07	6.10	7.27	9.05	10.6
12	1.53	2.33	3.00	3.73	4.82	5.76	6.80	8.38	9.74
13	1.51	2.28	2.92	3.60	4.62	5.48	6.44	7.86	9.07
14	1.50	2.24	2.85	3.50	4.46	5.26	6.14	7.44	8.53
15	1.48	2.21	2.79	3.41	4.32	5.07	5.89	7.09	8.10
16	1.47	2.18	2.74	3.34	4.20	4.91	5.68	6.80	7.74
17	1.46	2.15	2.70	3.28	4.10	4.78	5.51	6.56	7.43
18	1.45	2.13	2.66	3.22	4.01	4.66	5.36	6.35	7.18
19	1.44	2.11	2.63	3.17	3.94	4.56	5.23	6.18	6.95
20	1.44	2.09	2.60	3.13	3.87	4.47	5.11	6.02	6.76
21	1.43	2.08	2.57	3.09	3.81	4.39	5.01	5.88	6.59
22	1.42	2.06	2.55	3.05	3.76	4.32	4.92	5.76	6.44
23	1.42	2.05	2.53	3.02	3.71	4.26	4.84	5.65	6.30
24	1.41	2.04	2.51	2.99	3.67	4.20	4.76	5.55	6.18
25	1.41	2.02	2.49	2.97	3.63	4.15	4.70	5.46	6.07
26	1.41	2.01	2.47	2.94	3.59	4.10	4.64	5.38	5.98
27	1.40	2.00	2.46	2.92	3.56	4.06	4.58	5.31	5.89
28	1.40	2.00	2.45	2.90	3.53	4.02	4.53	5.24	5.80
29	1.40	1.99	2.43	2.88	3.50	3.98	4.48	5.18	5.73
30	1.39	1.98	2.42	2.87	3.47	3.95	4.44	5.12	5.66
35	1.38	1.95	2.37	2.80	3.37	3.81	4.27	4.89	5.39
40	1.37	1.93	2.34	2.74	3.29	3.71	4.14	4.73	5.19
45	1.36	1.91	2.31	2.70	3.23	3.64	4.05	4.61	5.04
50	1.36	1.90	2.29	2.67	3.19	3.58	3.98	4.51	4.93
60	1.35	1.87	2.25	2.63	3.12	3.49	3.87	4.37	4.76
70	1.34	1.86	2.23	2.59	3.07	3.43	3.79	4.28	4.64
80	1.34	1.85	2.21	2.57	3.04	3.39	3.74	4.20	4.56
90	1.33	1.84	2.20	2.55	3.01	3.35	3.70	4.15	4.50
100	1.33	1.83	2.19	2.54	2.99	3.33	3.66	4.11	4.45
200	1.32	1.80	2.14	2.47	2.89	3.21	3.52	3.92	4.22
500	1.31	1.79	2.12	2.43	2.84	3.14	3.43	3.81	4.10
∞	1.31	1.77	2.10	2.41	2.80	3.09	3.37	3.74	4.02

Table B.4 *Continued*

					Numerator df = 7				
α(l)	0.25	0.10	0.05	0.025	0.01	0.005	0.0025	0.001	0.0005
Denom df									
1	9.10	58.9	237.	948.	5930.	23700.	94900.	$6 \cdot 10^5$	$2 \cdot 10^6$
2	3.34	9.35	19.4	39.4	99.4	199.	399.	999.	2000.
3	2.43	5.27	8.89	14.6	27.7	44.4	71.0	132.	209.
4	2.08	3.98	6.09	9.07	15.0	21.6	31.0	49.7	70.7
5	1.89	3.37	4.88	6.85	10.5	14.2	19.1	28.2	37.6
6	1.78	3.01	4.21	5.70	8.26	10.8	14.0	19.5	24.9
7	1.70	2.78	3.79	4.99	6.99	8.89	11.2	15.0	18.7
8	1.64	2.62	3.50	4.53	6.18	7.69	9.49	12.4	15.1
9	1.60	2.51	3.29	4.20	5.61	6.88	8.36	10.7	12.8
10	1.57	2.41	3.14	3.95	5.20	6.30	7.56	9.52	11.2
11	1.54	2.34	3.01	3.76	4.89	5.86	6.97	8.66	10.1
12	1.52	2.28	2.91	3.61	4.64	5.52	6.51	8.00	9.28
13	1.50	2.23	2.83	3.48	4.44	5.25	6.15	7.49	8.63
14	1.49	2.19	2.76	3.38	4.28	5.03	5.86	7.08	8.11
15	1.47	2.16	2.71	3.29	4.14	4.85	5.62	6.74	7.68
16	1.46	2.13	2.66	3.22	4.03	4.69	5.41	6.46	7.33
17	1.45	2.10	2.61	3.16	3.93	4.56	5.24	6.22	7.04
18	1.44	2.08	2.58	3.10	3.84	4.44	5.09	6.02	6.78
19	1.43	2.06	2.54	3.05	3.77	4.34	4.96	5.85	6.57
20	1.43	2.04	2.51	3.01	3.70	4.26	4.85	5.69	6.38
21	1.42	2.02	2.49	2.97	3.64	4.18	4.75	5.56	6.21
22	1.41	2.01	2.46	2.93	3.59	4.11	4.66	5.44	6.07
23	1.41	1.99	2.44	2.90	3.54	4.05	4.58	5.33	5.94
24	1.40	1.98	2.42	2.87	3.50	3.99	4.51	5.23	5.82
25	1.40	1.97	2.40	2.85	3.46	3.94	4.44	5.15	5.71
26	1.39	1.96	2.39	2.82	3.42	3.89	4.38	5.07	5.62
27	1.39	1.95	2.37	2.80	3.39	3.85	4.33	5.00	5.53
28	1.39	1.94	2.36	2.78	3.36	3.81	4.28	4.93	5.45
29	1.38	1.93	2.35	2.76	3.33	3.77	4.24	4.87	5.38
30	1.38	1.93	2.33	2.75	3.30	3.74	4.19	4.82	5.31
35	1.37	1.90	2.29	2.68	3.20	3.61	4.02	4.59	5.04
40	1.36	1.87	2.25	2.62	3.12	3.51	3.90	4.44	4.85
45	1.35	1.85	2.22	2.58	3.07	3.43	3.81	4.32	4.71
50	1.34	1.84	2.20	2.55	3.02	3.38	3.74	4.22	4.60
60	1.33	1.82	2.17	2.51	2.95	3.29	3.63	4.09	4.44
70	1.33	1.80	2.14	2.47	2.91	3.23	3.56	3.99	4.32
80	1.32	1.79	2.13	2.45	2.87	3.19	3.50	3.92	4.24
90	1.32	1.78	2.11	2.43	2.84	3.15	3.46	3.87	4.18
100	1.32	1.78	2.10	2.42	2.82	3.13	3.43	3.83	4.13
200	1.30	1.75	2.06	2.35	2.73	3.01	3.29	3.65	3.92
500	1.30	1.73	2.03	2.31	2.68	2.94	3.20	3.54	3.80
∞	1.29	1.72	2.01	2.29	2.64	2.90	3.15	3.47	3.72

Table B.4   *Continued*

				Numerator df = 8					
α(↓)	0.25	0.10	0.05	0.025	0.01	0.005	0.0025	0.001	0.0005
Denom df									
1	9.19	59.4	239.	957.	5980.	23900.	95700.	$6 \cdot 10^5$	$2 \cdot 10^6$
2	3.35	9.37	19.4	39.4	99.4	199.	399.	999.	2000.
3	2.44	5.25	8.85	14.5	27.5	44.1	70.5	131.	208.
4	2.08	3.95	6.04	8.98	14.8	21.4	30.6	49.0	69.7
5	1.89	3.34	4.82	6.76	10.3	14.0	18.8	27.6	36.9
6	1.78	2.98	4.15	5.60	8.10	10.6	13.7	19.0	24.3
7	1.70	2.75	3.73	4.90	6.84	8.68	10.9	14.6	18.2
8	1.64	2.59	3.44	4.43	6.03	7.50	9.24	12.0	14.6
9	1.60	2.47	3.23	4.10	5.47	6.69	8.12	10.4	12.4
10	1.56	2.38	3.07	3.85	5.06	6.12	7.33	9.20	10.9
11	1.53	2.30	2.95	3.66	4.74	5.68	6.74	8.35	9.76
12	1.51	2.24	2.85	3.51	4.50	5.35	6.29	7.71	8.94
13	1.49	2.20	2.77	3.39	4.30	5.08	5.93	7.21	8.29
14	1.48	2.15	2.70	3.29	4.14	4.86	5.64	6.80	7.78
15	1.46	2.12	2.64	3.20	4.00	4.67	5.40	6.47	7.37
16	1.45	2.09	2.59	3.12	3.89	4.52	5.20	6.19	7.02
17	1.44	2.06	2.55	3.06	3.79	4.39	5.03	5.96	6.73
18	1.43	2.04	2.51	3.01	3.71	4.28	4.89	5.76	6.48
19	1.42	2.02	2.48	2.96	3.63	4.18	4.76	5.59	6.27
20	1.42	2.00	2.45	2.91	3.56	4.09	4.65	5.44	6.09
21	1.41	1.98	2.42	2.87	3.51	4.01	4.55	5.31	5.92
22	1.40	1.97	2.40	2.84	3.45	3.94	4.46	5.19	5.78
23	1.40	1.95	2.37	2.81	3.41	3.88	4.38	5.09	5.65
24	1.39	1.94	2.36	2.78	3.36	3.83	4.31	4.99	5.54
25	1.39	1.93	2.34	2.75	3.32	3.78	4.25	4.91	5.43
26	1.38	1.92	2.32	2.73	3.29	3.73	4.19	4.83	5.34
27	1.38	1.91	2.31	2.71	3.26	3.69	4.14	4.76	5.25
28	1.38	1.90	2.29	2.69	3.23	3.65	4.09	4.69	5.18
29	1.37	1.89	2.28	2.67	3.20	3.61	4.04	4.64	5.11
30	1.37	1.88	2.27	2.65	3.17	3.58	4.00	4.58	5.04
35	1.36	1.85	2.22	2.58	3.07	3.45	3.83	4.36	4.78
40	1.35	1.83	2.18	2.53	2.99	3.35	3.71	4.21	4.59
45	1.34	1.81	2.15	2.49	2.94	3.28	3.62	4.09	4.45
50	1.33	1.80	2.13	2.46	2.89	3.22	3.55	4.00	4.34
60	1.32	1.77	2.10	2.41	2.82	3.13	3.45	3.86	4.19
70	1.32	1.76	2.07	2.38	2.78	3.08	3.37	3.77	4.08
80	1.31	1.75	2.06	2.35	2.74	3.03	3.32	3.70	4.00
90	1.31	1.74	2.04	2.34	2.72	3.00	3.28	3.65	3.94
100	1.30	1.73	2.03	2.32	2.69	2.97	3.25	3.61	3.89
200	1.29	1.70	1.98	2.26	2.60	2.86	3.11	3.43	3.68
500	1.28	1.68	1.96	2.22	2.55	2.79	3.03	3.33	3.56
∞	1.28	1.67	1.94	2.19	2.51	2.74	2.97	3.27	3.48

Table B.4 *Continued*

					Numerator df = 9				
$\alpha(\mid)$	0.25	0.10	0.05	0.025	0.01	0.005	0.0025	0.001	0.0005
Denom df									
1	9.26	59.9	241.	963.	6020.	24100.	96400.	$6 \cdot 10^5$	$2 \cdot 10^6$
2	3.37	9.38	19.4	39.4	99.4	199.	399.	999.	2000.
3	2.44	5.24	8.81	14.5	27.3	43.9	70.1	130.	207.
4	2.08	3.94	6.00	8.90	14.7	21.1	30.3	48.5	69.0
5	1.89	3.32	4.77	6.68	10.2	13.8	18.5	27.2	36.3
6	1.77	2.96	4.10	5.52	7.98	10.4	13.4	18.7	23.9
7	1.69	2.72	3.68	4.82	6.72	8.51	10.7	14.3	17.8
8	1.63	2.56	3.39	4.36	5.91	7.34	9.03	11.8	14.3
9	1.59	2.44	3.18	4.03	5.35	6.54	7.92	10.1	12.1
10	1.56	2.35	3.02	3.78	4.94	5.97	7.14	8.96	10.6
11	1.53	2.27	2.90	3.59	4.63	5.54	6.56	8.12	9.48
12	1.51	2.21	2.80	3.44	4.39	5.20	6.11	7.48	8.66
13	1.49	2.16	2.71	3.31	4.19	4.94	5.76	6.98	8.03
14	1.47	2.12	2.65	3.21	4.03	4.72	5.47	6.58	7.52
15	1.46	2.09	2.59	3.12	3.89	4.54	5.23	6.26	7.11
16	1.44	2.06	2.54	3.05	3.78	4.38	5.04	5.98	6.77
17	1.43	2.03	2.49	2.98	3.68	4.25	4.87	5.75	6.49
18	1.42	2.02	2.46	2.93	3.60	4.14	4.72	5.56	6.24
19	1.41	1.98	2.42	2.88	3.52	4.04	4.60	5.39	6.03
20	1.41	1.96	2.39	2.84	3.46	3.96	4.49	5.24	5.85
21	1.40	1.95	2.37	2.80	3.40	3.88	4.39	5.11	5.69
22	1.39	1.93	2.34	2.76	3.35	3.81	4.30	4.99	5.55
23	1.39	1.92	2.32	2.73	3.30	3.75	4.22	4.89	5.43
24	1.38	1.91	2.30	2.70	3.26	3.69	4.15	4.80	5.31
25	1.38	1.89	2.28	2.68	3.22	3.64	4.09	4.71	5.21
26	1.37	1.88	2.27	2.65	3.18	3.60	4.03	4.64	5.12
27	1.37	1.87	2.25	2.63	3.15	3.56	3.98	4.57	5.04
28	1.37	1.87	2.24	2.61	3.12	3.52	3.93	4.50	4.96
29	1.36	1.86	2.22	2.59	3.09	3.48	3.89	4.45	4.89
30	1.36	1.85	2.21	2.57	3.07	3.45	3.85	4.39	4.82
35	1.35	1.82	2.16	2.50	2.96	3.32	3.68	4.18	4.57
40	1.34	1.79	2.12	2.45	2.89	3.22	3.56	4.02	4.38
45	1.33	1.77	2.10	2.41	2.83	3.15	3.47	3.91	4.25
50	1.32	1.76	2.07	2.38	2.78	3.09	3.40	3.82	4.14
60	1.31	1.74	2.04	2.33	2.72	3.01	3.30	3.69	3.98
70	1.31	1.72	2.02	2.30	2.67	2.95	3.23	3.60	3.88
80	1.30	1.71	2.00	2.28	2.64	2.91	3.17	3.53	3.80
90	1.30	1.70	1.99	2.26	2.61	2.87	3.13	3.48	3.74
100	1.29	1.69	1.97	2.24	2.59	2.85	3.10	3.44	3.69
200	1.28	1.66	1.93	2.18	2.50	2.73	2.96	3.26	3.49
500	1.27	1.64	1.90	2.14	2.44	2.66	2.88	3.16	3.37
∞	1.27	1.63	1.88	2.11	2.41	2.62	2.83	3.10	3.30

Table B.4 *Continued*

				Numerator df = 10					
$\alpha(1)$	0.25	0.10	0.05	0.025	0.01	0.005	0.0025	0.001	0.0005
Denom df									
1	9.32	60.2	242.	969.	6060.	24200.	96900.	$6 \cdot 10^5$	$2 \cdot 10^6$
2	3.38	9.39	19.4	39.4	99.4	199.	399.	999.	2000.
3	2.44	5.23	8.79	14.4	27.2	43.7	69.8	129.	206.
4	2.08	3.92	5.96	8.84	14.5	21.0	30.0	48.1	68.3
5	1.89	3.30	4.74	6.62	10.1	13.6	18.3	26.9	35.9
6	1.77	2.94	4.06	5.46	7.87	10.3	13.2	18.4	23.5
7	1.69	2.70	3.64	4.76	6.62	8.38	10.5	14.1	17.5
8	1.63	2.54	3.35	4.30	5.81	7.21	8.87	11.5	14.0
9	1.59	2.42	3.14	3.96	5.26	6.42	7.77	9.89	11.8
10	1.55	2.32	2.98	3.72	4.85	5.85	6.99	8.75	10.3
11	1.52	2.25	2.85	3.53	4.54	5.42	6.41	7.92	9.24
12	1.50	2.19	2.75	3.37	4.30	5.09	5.97	7.29	8.43
13	1.48	2.14	2.67	3.25	4.10	4.82	5.62	6.80	7.81
14	1.46	2.10	2.60	3.15	3.94	4.60	5.33	6.40	7.31
15	1.45	2.06	2.54	3.06	3.80	4.42	5.10	6.08	6.91
16	1.44	2.03	2.49	2.99	3.69	4.27	4.90	5.81	6.57
17	1.43	2.00	2.45	2.92	3.59	4.14	4.73	5.58	6.29
18	1.42	1.98	2.41	2.87	3.51	4.03	4.59	5.39	6.05
19	1.41	1.96	2.38	2.82	3.43	3.93	4.46	5.22	5.81
20	1.40	1.94	2.35	2.77	3.37	3.85	4.35	5.08	5.66
21	1.39	1.92	2.32	2.73	3.31	3.77	4.26	4.95	5.50
22	1.39	1.90	2.30	2.70	3.26	3.70	4.17	4.83	5.36
23	1.38	1.89	2.27	2.67	3.21	3.64	4.09	4.73	5.24
24	1.38	1.88	2.25	2.64	3.17	3.59	4.03	4.64	5.13
25	1.37	1.87	2.24	2.61	3.13	3.54	3.96	4.56	5.03
26	1.37	1.86	2.22	2.59	3.09	3.49	3.91	4.48	4.94
27	1.36	1.85	2.20	2.57	3.06	3.45	3.85	4.41	4.86
28	1.36	1.84	2.19	2.55	3.03	3.41	3.81	4.35	4.78
29	1.35	1.83	2.18	2.53	3.00	3.38	3.76	4.29	4.71
30	1.35	1.82	2.16	2.51	2.98	3.34	3.72	4.24	4.65
35	1.34	1.79	2.11	2.44	2.88	3.21	3.56	4.03	4.39
40	1.33	1.76	2.08	2.39	2.80	3.12	3.44	3.87	4.21
45	1.32	1.74	2.05	2.35	2.74	3.04	3.35	3.76	4.08
50	1.31	1.73	2.03	2.32	2.70	2.99	3.28	3.67	3.97
60	1.30	1.71	1.99	2.27	2.63	2.90	3.18	3.54	3.82
70	1.30	1.69	1.97	2.24	2.59	2.85	3.11	3.45	3.71
80	1.29	1.68	1.95	2.21	2.55	2.80	3.05	3.39	3.64
90	1.29	1.67	1.94	2.19	2.52	2.77	3.01	3.34	3.58
100	1.28	1.66	1.93	2.18	2.50	2.74	2.98	3.30	3.53
200	1.27	1.63	1.88	2.11	2.41	2.63	2.84	3.12	3.33
500	1.26	1.61	1.85	2.07	2.36	2.56	2.76	3.02	3.22
∞	1.25	1.60	1.83	2.05	2.32	2.52	2.71	2.96	3.14

Table B.4 *Continued*

				Numerator df = 12					
α(l)	0.25	0.10	0.05	0.025	0.01	0.005	0.0025	0.001	0.0005
Denom df									
1	9.41	60.7	244.	977.	6110.	24400.	97700.	$6 \cdot 10^5$	$2 \cdot 10^6$
2	3.39	9.41	19.4	39.4	99.4	199.	399.	999.	2000.
3	2.45	5.22	8.74	14.3	27.1	43.4	69.3	128.	204.
4	2.08	3.90	5.91	8.75	14.4	20.7	29.7	47.4	67.4
5	1.89	3.27	4.68	6.52	9.89	13.4	18.0	26.4	35.2
6	1.77	2.90	4.00	5.37	7.72	10.0	12.9	18.0	23.0
7	1.68	2.67	3.57	4.67	6.47	8.18	10.3	13.7	17.0
8	1.62	2.50	3.28	4.20	5.67	7.01	8.61	11.2	13.6
9	1.58	2.38	3.07	3.87	5.11	6.23	7.52	9.57	11.4
10	1.54	2.28	2.91	3.62	4.71	5.66	6.75	8.45	9.94
11	1.51	2.21	2.79	3.43	4.40	5.24	6.18	7.63	8.88
12	1.49	2.15	2.69	3.28	4.16	4.91	5.74	7.00	8.09
13	1.47	2.10	2.60	3.15	3.96	4.64	5.40	6.52	7.48
14	1.45	2.05	2.53	3.05	3.80	4.43	5.12	6.13	6.99
15	1.44	2.02	2.48	2.96	3.67	4.25	4.88	5.81	6.59
16	1.43	1.99	2.42	2.89	3.55	4.10	4.69	5.55	6.26
17	1.41	1.96	2.38	2.82	3.46	3.97	4.52	5.32	5.98
18	1.40	1.93	2.34	2.77	3.37	3.86	4.38	5.13	5.75
19	1.40	1.91	2.31	2.72	3.30	3.76	4.26	4.97	5.55
20	1.39	1.89	2.28	2.68	3.23	3.68	4.15	4.82	5.37
21	1.38	1.87	2.25	2.64	3.17	3.60	4.06	4.70	5.21
22	1.37	1.86	2.23	2.60	3.12	3.54	3.97	4.58	5.08
23	1.37	1.84	2.20	2.57	3.07	3.47	3.89	4.48	4.96
24	1.36	1.83	2.18	2.54	3.03	3.42	3.83	4.39	4.85
25	1.36	1.82	2.16	2.51	2.99	3.37	3.76	4.31	4.75
26	1.35	1.81	2.15	2.49	2.96	3.33	3.71	4.24	4.66
27	1.35	1.80	2.13	2.47	2.93	3.28	3.66	4.17	4.58
28	1.34	1.79	2.12	2.45	2.90	3.25	3.61	4.11	4.51
29	1.34	1.78	2.10	2.43	2.87	3.21	3.56	4.05	4.44
30	1.34	1.77	2.09	2.41	2.84	3.18	3.52	4.00	4.38
35	1.32	1.74	2.04	2.34	2.74	3.05	3.36	3.79	4.13
40	1.31	1.71	2.00	2.29	2.66	2.95	3.25	3.64	3.95
45	1.30	1.70	1.97	2.25	2.61	2.88	3.16	3.53	3.82
50	1.30	1.68	1.95	2.22	2.56	2.82	3.09	3.44	3.71
60	1.29	1.66	1.92	2.17	2.50	2.74	2.99	3.32	3.57
70	1.28	1.64	1.89	2.14	2.45	2.68	2.92	3.23	3.46
80	1.27	1.63	1.88	2.11	2.42	2.64	2.87	3.16	3.39
90	1.27	1.62	1.86	2.09	2.39	2.61	2.83	3.11	3.33
100	1.27	1.61	1.85	2.08	2.37	2.58	2.80	3.07	3.28
200	1.25	1.58	1.80	2.01	2.27	2.47	2.66	2.90	3.09
500	1.24	1.56	1.77	1.97	2.22	2.40	2.58	2.81	2.97
∞	1.24	1.55	1.75	1.94	2.18	2.36	2.53	2.74	2.90

Table B.4 *Continued*

					Numerator df = 14				
α(↓)	0.25	0.10	0.05	0.025	0.01	0.005	0.0025	0.001	0.0005
Denom df									
1	9.47	61.1	245.	983.	6140.	24600.	98300.	$6 \cdot 10^5$	$2 \cdot 10^6$
2	3.41	9.42	19.4	39.4	99.4	199.	399.	999.	2000.
3	2.45	5.20	8.71	14.3	26.9	43.2	69.0	128.	203.
4	2.08	3.88	5.87	8.68	14.2	20.5	29.4	46.9	66.8
5	1.89	3.25	4.64	6.46	9.77	13.2	17.8	26.1	34.7
6	1.76	2.88	3.96	5.30	7.60	9.88	12.7	17.7	22.6
7	1.68	2.64	3.53	4.60	6.36	8.03	10.1	13.4	16.6
8	1.62	2.48	3.24	4.13	5.56	6.87	8.43	10.9	13.3
9	1.57	2.35	3.03	3.80	5.01	6.09	7.35	9.33	11.1
10	1.54	2.26	2.86	3.55	4.60	5.53	6.58	8.22	9.67
11	1.51	2.18	2.74	3.36	4.29	5.10	6.02	7.41	8.62
12	1.48	2.12	2.64	3.21	4.05	4.77	5.58	6.79	7.84
13	1.46	2.07	2.55	3.08	3.86	4.51	5.24	6.31	7.23
14	1.44	2.02	2.48	2.98	3.70	4.30	4.96	5.93	6.75
15	1.43	1.99	2.42	2.89	3.56	4.12	4.73	5.62	6.36
16	1.42	1.95	2.37	2.82	3.45	3.97	4.54	5.35	6.03
17	1.41	1.93	2.33	2.75	3.35	3.84	4.37	5.13	5.76
18	1.40	1.90	2.29	2.70	3.27	3.73	4.23	4.94	5.53
19	1.39	1.88	2.26	2.65	3.19	3.64	4.11	4.78	5.33
20	1.38	1.86	2.22	2.60	3.13	3.55	4.00	4.64	5.15
21	1.37	1.84	2.20	2.56	3.07	3.48	3.91	4.51	5.00
22	1.36	1.83	2.17	2.53	3.02	3.41	3.82	4.40	4.87
23	1.36	1.81	2.15	2.50	2.97	3.35	3.75	4.30	4.75
24	1.35	1.80	2.13	2.47	2.93	3.30	3.68	4.21	4.64
25	1.35	1.79	2.11	2.44	2.89	3.25	3.62	4.13	4.54
26	1.34	1.77	2.09	2.42	2.86	3.20	3.56	4.06	4.46
27	1.34	1.76	2.08	2.39	2.82	3.16	3.51	3.99	4.38
28	1.33	1.75	2.06	2.37	2.79	3.12	3.46	3.93	4.30
29	1.33	1.75	2.05	2.36	2.77	3.09	3.42	3.88	4.24
30	1.33	1.74	2.04	2.34	2.74	3.06	3.38	3.82	4.18
35	1.31	1.70	1.99	2.27	2.64	2.93	3.22	3.62	3.93
40	1.30	1.68	1.95	2.21	2.56	2.83	3.10	3.47	3.76
45	1.29	1.66	1.92	2.17	2.51	2.76	3.02	3.36	3.63
50	1.28	1.64	1.89	2.14	2.46	2.70	2.95	3.27	3.52
60	1.27	1.62	1.86	2.09	2.39	2.62	2.85	3.15	3.38
70	1.27	1.60	1.84	2.06	2.35	2.56	2.78	3.06	3.28
80	1.26	1.59	1.82	2.03	2.31	2.52	2.73	3.00	3.20
90	1.26	1.58	1.80	2.02	2.29	2.49	2.69	2.95	3.14
100	1.25	1.57	1.79	2.00	2.27	2.46	2.65	2.91	3.10
200	1.24	1.54	1.74	1.93	2.17	2.35	2.52	2.74	2.91
500	1.23	1.52	1.71	1.89	2.12	2.28	2.44	2.64	2.79
∞	1.22	1.50	1.69	1.87	2.08	2.24	2.39	2.58	2.72

Table B.4   *Continued*

				Numerator df = 16					
α(l)	0.25	0.10	0.05	0.025	0.01	0.005	0.0025	0.001	0.0005
Denom df									
1	9.52	61.3	246.	987.	6170.	24700.	98700.	$6 \cdot 10^5$	$2 \cdot 10^6$
2	3.41	9.43	19.4	39.4	99.4	199.	399.	999.	2000.
3	2.46	5.20	8.69	14.2	26.8	43.0	68.7	127.	202.
4	2.08	3.86	5.84	8.63	14.2	20.4	29.2	46.6	66.2
5	1.88	3.23	4.60	6.40	9.68	13.1	17.6	25.8	34.3
6	1.76	2.86	3.92	5.24	7.52	9.76	12.6	17.4	22.3
7	1.68	2.62	3.49	4.54	6.28	7.91	9.91	13.2	16.4
8	1.62	2.45	3.20	4.08	5.48	6.76	8.29	10.8	13.0
9	1.57	2.33	2.99	3.74	4.92	5.98	7.21	9.15	10.9
10	1.53	2.23	2.83	3.50	4.52	5.42	6.45	8.05	9.46
11	1.50	2.16	2.70	3.30	4.21	5.00	5.89	7.24	8.43
12	1.48	2.09	2.60	3.15	3.97	4.67	5.46	6.63	7.65
13	1.46	2.04	2.51	3.03	3.78	4.41	5.11	6.16	7.05
14	1.44	2.00	2.44	2.92	3.62	4.20	4.84	5.78	6.57
15	1.42	1.96	2.38	2.84	3.49	4.02	4.61	5.46	6.18
16	1.41	1.93	2.33	2.76	3.37	3.87	4.42	5.20	5.86
17	1.40	1.90	2.29	2.70	3.27	3.75	4.25	4.99	5.59
18	1.39	1.87	2.25	2.64	3.19	3.64	4.11	4.80	5.36
19	1.38	1.85	2.21	2.59	3.12	3.54	3.99	4.64	5.16
20	1.37	1.83	2.18	2.55	3.05	3.46	3.89	4.49	4.99
21	1.36	1.81	2.16	2.51	2.99	3.38	3.79	4.37	4.84
22	1.36	1.80	2.13	2.47	2.94	3.31	3.71	4.26	4.71
23	1.35	1.78	2.11	2.44	2.89	3.25	3.63	4.16	4.59
24	1.34	1.77	2.09	2.41	2.85	3.20	3.56	4.07	4.48
25	1.34	1.76	2.07	2.38	2.81	3.15	3.50	3.99	4.39
26	1.33	1.75	2.05	2.36	2.78	3.11	3.45	3.92	4.30
27	1.33	1.74	2.04	2.34	2.75	3.07	3.40	3.86	4.22
28	1.32	1.73	2.02	2.32	2.72	3.03	3.35	3.80	4.15
29	1.32	1.72	2.01	2.30	2.69	2.99	3.31	3.74	4.08
30	1.32	1.71	1.99	2.28	2.66	2.96	3.27	3.69	4.02
35	1.30	1.67	1.94	2.21	2.56	2.83	3.11	3.48	3.78
40	1.29	1.65	1.90	2.15	2.48	2.74	2.99	3.34	3.61
45	1.28	1.63	1.87	2.11	2.43	2.66	2.90	3.23	3.48
50	1.27	1.61	1.85	2.08	2.38	2.61	2.84	3.14	3.38
60	1.26	1.59	1.82	2.03	2.31	2.53	2.74	3.02	3.23
70	1.26	1.57	1.79	2.00	2.27	2.47	2.67	2.93	3.13
80	1.25	1.56	1.77	1.97	2.23	2.43	2.62	2.87	3.06
90	1.25	1.55	1.76	1.95	2.21	2.39	2.58	2.82	3.00
100	1.24	1.54	1.75	1.94	2.19	2.37	2.55	2.78	2.96
200	1.23	1.51	1.69	1.87	2.09	2.25	2.41	2.61	2.76
500	1.22	1.49	1.66	1.83	2.04	2.19	2.33	2.52	2.65
∞	1.21	1.47	1.64	1.80	2.00	2.14	2.28	2.45	2.58

Table B.4 *Continued*

					Numerator df = 18				
α(ꟼ)	0.25	0.10	0.05	0.025	0.01	0.005	0.0025	0.001	0.0005
Denom df									
1	9.55	61.6	247.	990.	6190.	24800.	99100.	$6 \cdot 10^5$	$2 \cdot 10^6$
2	3.42	9.44	19.4	39.4	99.4	199.	399.	999.	2000.
3	2.46	5.19	8.67	14.2	26.8	42.9	68.5	127.	202.
4	2.08	3.85	5.82	8.59	14.1	20.3	29.0	46.3	65.8
5	1.88	3.22	4.58	6.36	9.61	13.0	17.4	25.6	34.0
6	1.76	2.85	3.90	5.20	7.45	9.66	12.4	17.3	22.0
7	1.67	2.61	3.47	4.50	6.21	7.83	9.79	13.1	16.2
8	1.61	2.44	3.17	4.03	5.41	6.68	8.18	10.6	12.8
9	1.56	2.31	2.96	3.70	4.86	5.90	7.11	9.01	10.7
10	1.53	2.22	2.80	3.45	4.46	5.34	6.35	7.91	9.30
11	1.50	2.14	2.67	3.26	4.15	4.92	5.79	7.11	8.27
12	1.47	2.08	2.57	3.11	3.91	4.59	5.36	6.51	7.50
13	1.45	2.02	2.48	2.98	3.72	4.33	5.02	6.03	6.90
14	1.43	1.98	2.41	2.88	3.56	4.12	4.74	5.66	6.43
15	1.42	1.94	2.35	2.79	3.42	3.95	4.51	5.35	6.04
16	1.40	1.91	2.30	2.72	3.31	3.80	4.32	5.09	5.72
17	1.39	1.88	2.26	2.65	3.21	3.67	4.16	4.87	5.45
18	1.38	1.85	2.22	2.60	3.13	3.56	4.02	4.68	5.23
19	1.37	1.83	2.18	2.55	3.05	3.46	3.90	4.52	5.03
20	1.36	1.81	2.15	2.50	2.99	3.38	3.79	4.38	4.86
21	1.36	1.79	2.12	2.46	2.93	3.31	3.70	4.26	4.71
22	1.35	1.78	2.10	2.43	2.88	3.24	3.62	4.15	4.58
23	1.34	1.76	2.08	2.39	2.83	3.18	3.54	4.05	4.46
24	1.34	1.75	2.05	2.36	2.79	3.12	3.47	3.96	4.35
25	1.33	1.74	2.04	2.34	2.75	3.08	3.41	3.88	4.26
26	1.33	1.72	2.02	2.31	2.72	3.03	3.36	3.81	4.17
27	1.32	1.71	2.00	2.29	2.68	2.99	3.31	3.75	4.10
28	1.32	1.70	1.99	2.27	2.65	2.95	3.26	3.69	4.02
29	1.31	1.69	1.97	2.25	2.63	2.92	3.22	3.63	3.96
30	1.31	1.69	1.96	2.23	2.60	2.89	3.18	3.58	3.90
35	1.29	1.65	1.91	2.16	2.50	2.76	3.02	3.38	3.66
40	1.28	1.62	1.87	2.11	2.42	2.66	2.90	3.23	3.49
45	1.27	1.60	1.84	2.07	2.36	2.59	2.82	3.12	3.36
50	1.27	1.59	1.81	2.03	2.32	2.53	2.75	3.04	3.26
60	1.26	1.56	1.78	1.98	2.25	2.45	2.65	2.91	3.11
70	1.25	1.55	1.75	1.95	2.20	2.39	2.58	2.83	3.01
80	1.24	1.53	1.73	1.92	2.17	2.35	2.53	2.76	2.94
90	1.24	1.52	1.72	1.91	2.14	2.32	2.49	2.71	2.88
100	1.23	1.52	1.71	1.89	2.12	2.29	2.46	2.68	2.84
200	1.22	1.48	1.66	1.82	2.03	2.18	2.32	2.51	2.65
500	1.21	1.46	1.62	1.78	1.97	2.11	2.24	2.41	2.54
∞	1.20	1.44	1.60	1.75	1.93	2.06	2.19	2.35	2.47

Table B.4   *Continued*

				Numerator df = 20					
$\alpha(\ |\ )$	0.25	0.10	0.05	0.025	0.01	0.005	0.0025	0.001	0.0005
Denom df									
1	9.58	61.7	248.	993.	6210.	24800.	99300.	$6 \cdot 10^5$	$2 \cdot 10^6$
2	3.43	9.44	19.4	39.4	99.4	199.	399.	999.	2000.
3	2.46	5.18	8.66	14.2	26.7	42.8	68.3	126.	201.
4	2.08	3.84	5.80	8.56	14.0	20.2	28.9	46.1	65.5
5	1.88	3.21	4.56	6.33	9.55	12.9	17.3	25.4	33.8
6	1.76	2.84	3.87	5.17	7.40	9.59	12.3	17.1	21.8
7	1.67	2.59	3.44	4.47	6.16	7.75	9.70	12.9	16.0
8	1.61	2.42	3.15	4.00	5.36	6.61	8.09	10.5	12.7
9	1.56	2.30	2.94	3.67	4.81	5.83	7.02	8.90	10.6
10	1.52	2.20	2.77	3.42	4.41	5.27	6.27	7.80	9.17
11	1.49	2.12	2.65	3.23	4.10	4.86	5.71	7.01	8.14
12	1.47	2.06	2.54	3.07	3.86	4.53	5.28	6.40	7.37
13	1.45	2.01	2.46	2.95	3.66	4.27	4.94	5.93	6.78
14	1.43	1.96	2.39	2.84	3.51	4.06	4.66	5.56	6.31
15	1.41	1.92	2.33	2.76	3.37	3.88	4.44	5.25	5.93
16	1.40	1.89	2.28	2.68	3.26	3.73	4.25	4.99	5.61
17	1.39	1.86	2.23	2.62	3.16	3.61	4.09	4.78	5.34
18	1.38	1.84	2.19	2.56	3.08	3.50	3.95	4.59	5.12
19	1.37	1.81	2.16	2.51	3.00	3.40	3.83	4.43	4.92
20	1.36	1.79	2.12	2.46	2.94	3.32	3.72	4.29	4.75
21	1.35	1.78	2.10	2.42	2.88	3.24	3.63	4.17	4.60
22	1.34	1.76	2.07	2.39	2.83	3.18	3.54	4.06	4.47
23	1.34	1.74	2.05	2.36	2.78	3.12	3.47	3.96	4.36
24	1.33	1.73	2.03	2.33	2.74	3.06	3.40	3.87	4.25
25	1.33	1.72	2.01	2.30	2.70	3.01	3.34	3.79	4.16
26	1.32	1.71	1.99	2.28	2.66	2.97	3.28	3.72	4.07
27	1.32	1.70	1.97	2.25	2.63	2.93	3.23	3.66	3.99
28	1.31	1.69	1.96	2.23	2.60	2.89	3.19	3.60	3.92
29	1.31	1.68	1.94	2.21	2.57	2.86	3.14	3.54	3.86
30	1.30	1.67	1.93	2.20	2.55	2.82	3.11	3.49	3.80
35	1.29	1.63	1.88	2.12	2.44	2.69	2.95	3.29	3.56
40	1.28	1.61	1.84	2.07	2.37	2.60	2.83	3.14	3.39
45	1.27	1.58	1.81	2.03	2.31	2.53	2.74	3.04	3.26
50	1.26	1.57	1.78	1.99	2.27	2.47	2.68	2.95	3.16
60	1.25	1.54	1.75	1.94	2.20	2.39	2.58	2.83	3.02
70	1.24	1.53	1.72	1.91	2.15	2.33	2.51	2.74	2.92
80	1.23	1.51	1.70	1.88	2.12	2.29	2.46	2.68	2.85
90	1.23	1.50	1.69	1.86	2.09	2.25	2.42	2.63	2.79
100	1.23	1.49	1.68	1.85	2.07	2.23	2.38	2.59	2.75
200	1.21	1.46	1.62	1.78	1.97	2.11	2.25	2.42	2.56
500	1.20	1.44	1.59	1.74	1.92	2.04	2.17	2.33	2.45
∞	1.19	1.42	1.57	1.71	1.88	2.00	2.12	2.27	2.37

Table B.4 *Continued*

				Numerator df = ∞					
α(l)	0.25	0.10	0.05	0.025	0.01	0.005	0.0025	0.001	0.0005
Denom df									
1	9.85	63.3	254.	1020.	6370.	25500.	$1 \cdot 10^5$	$6 \cdot 10^5$	$3 \cdot 10^6$
2	3.48	9.49	19.5	39.5	99.5	199.	399.	999..	2000.
3	2.47	5.13	8.53	13.9	26.1	41.8	66.8	123.	196.
4	2.08	3.76	5.63	8.26	13.5	19.3	27.6	44.0	62.6
5	1.87	3.11	4.37	6.02	9.02	12.1	16.3	23.8	31.6
6	1.74	2.72	3.67	4.85	6.88	8.88	11.4	15.7	20.0
7	1.65	2.47	3.23	4.14	5.65	7.08	8.81	11.7	14.4
8	1.58	2.29	2.93	3.67	4.86	5.95	7.25	9.33	11.3
9	1.53	2.16	2.71	3.33	4.31	5.19	6.21	7.81	9.26
10	1.48	2.06	2.54	3.08	3.91	4.64	5.47	6.76	7.91
11	1.45	1.97	2.40	2.88	3.60	4.23	4.93	6.00	6.93
12	1.42	1.90	2.30	2.72	3.36	3.90	4.51	5.42	6.20
13	1.40	1.85	2.21	2.60	3.17	3.65	4.18	4.97	5.64
14	1.38	1.80	2.13	2.49	3.00	3.44	3.91	4.60	5.19
15	1.36	1.76	2.07	2.40	2.87	3.26	3.69	4.31	4.83
16	1.34	1.72	2.01	2.32	2.75	3.11	3.50	4.06	4.52
17	1.33	1.69	1.96	2.25	2.65	2.98	3.34	3.85	4.27
18	1.32	1.66	1.92	2.19	2.57	2.87	3.20	3.67	4.05
19	1.30	1.63	1.88	2.13	2.49	2.78	3.08	3.51	3.87
20	1.29	1.61	1.84	2.09	2.42	2.69	2.97	3.38	3.71
21	1.28	1.59	1.81	2.04	2.36	2.61	2.88	3.26	3.56
22	1.28	1.57	1.78	2.00	2.31	2.55	2.80	3.15	3.43
23	1.27	1.55	1.76	1.97	2.26	2.48	2.72	3.05	3.32
24	1.26	1.53	1.73	1.94	2.21	2.43	2.65	2.97	3.22
25	1.25	1.52	1.71	1.91	2.17	2.38	2.59	2.89	3.13
26	1.25	1.50	1.69	1.88	2.13	2.33	2.54	2.82	3.05
27	1.24	1.49	1.67	1.85	2.10	2.29	2.48	2.75	2.97
28	1.24	1.48	1.65	1.83	2.06	2.25	2.44	2.69	2.90
29	1.23	1.47	1.64	1.81	2.03	2.21	2.39	2.64	2.84
30	1.23	1.46	1.62	1.79	2.01	2.18	2.35	2.59	2.78
35	1.20	1.41	1.56	1.70	1.89	2.04	2.18	2.38	2.54
40	1.19	1.38	1.51	1.64	1.80	1.93	2.06	2.23	2.37
45	1.18	1.35	1.47	1.59	1.74	1.85	1.97	2.12	2.23
50	1.16	1.33	1.44	1.55	1.68	1.79	1.89	2.03	2.13
60	1.15	1.29	1.39	1.48	1.60	1.69	1.78	1.89	1.98
70	1.13	1.27	1.35	1.44	1.54	1.62	1.69	1.79	1.87
80	1.12	1.24	1.32	1.40	1.49	1.56	1.63	1.72	1.79
90	1.12	1.23	1.30	1.37	1.46	1.52	1.58	1.66	1.72
100	1.11	1.21	1.28	1.35	1.43	1.49	1.54	1.62	1.67
200	1.07	1.14	1.19	1.23	1.28	1.31	1.35	1.39	1.42
500	1.05	1.09	1.11	1.14	1.16	1.18	1.20	1.23	1.24
∞	1.00	1.00	1.00	1.00	1.00	1.00	1.00	1.00	1.00

Table B.5   Critical values of Spearman's correlation coefficient*

$\alpha(2)$	0.50	0.20	0.10	0.05	0.02	0.01	0.005	0.002	0.001
$\alpha(1)$	0.25	0.10	0.05	0.025	0.01	0.005	0.0025	0.001	0.0005
n									
4	0.600	1.000	1.000						
5	0.500	0.800	0.900	1.000	1.000				
6	0.371	0.657	0.829	0.886	0.943	1.000	1.000		
7	0.321	0.571	0.714	0.786	0.893	0.929	0.964	1.000	1.000
8	0.310	0.524	0.643	0.738	0.833	0.881	0.905	0.952	0.976
9	0.267	0.483	0.600	0.700	0.783	0.833	0.867	0.917	0.933
10	0.248	0.455	0.564	0.648	0.745	0.794	0.830	0.879	0.903
11	0.236	0.427	0.536	0.618	0.709	0.755	0.800	0.845	0.873
12	0.217	0.406	0.503	0.587	0.678	0.727	0.769	0.818	0.846
13	0.209	0.385	0.484	0.560	0.648	0.703	0.747	0.791	0.824
14	0.200	0.367	0.464	0.538	0.626	0.679	0.723	0.771	0.802
15	0.189	0.354	0.446	0.521	0.604	0.654	0.700	0.750	0.779
16	0.182	0.341	0.429	0.503	0.582	0.635	0.679	0.729	0.762
17	0.176	0.328	0.414	0.485	0.566	0.615	0.662	0.713	0.748
18	0.170	0.317	0.401	0.472	0.550	0.600	0.643	0.695	0.728
19	0.165	0.309	0.391	0.460	0.535	0.584	0.628	0.677	0.712
20	0.161	0.299	0.380	0.447	0.520	0.570	0.612	0.662	0.696
21	0.156	0.292	0.370	0.435	0.508	0.556	0.599	0.648	0.681
22	0.152	0.284	0.361	0.425	0.496	0.544	0.586	0.634	0.667
23	0.148	0.278	0.353	0.415	0.486	0.532	0.573	0.622	0.654
24	0.144	0.271	0.344	0.406	0.476	0.521	0.562	0.610	0.642
25	0.142	0.265	0.337	0.398	0.466	0.511	0.551	0.598	0.630
26	0.138	0.259	0.331	0.390	0.457	0.501	0.541	0.587	0.619
27	0.136	0.255	0.324	0.382	0.448	0.491	0.531	0.577	0.608
28	0.133	0.250	0.317	0.375	0.440	0.483	0.522	0.567	0.598
29	0.130	0.245	0.312	0.368	0.433	0.475	0.513	0.558	0.589
30	0.128	0.240	0.306	0.362	0.425	0.467	0.504	0.549	0.580
35	0.118	0.222	0.283	0.335	0.394	0.433	0.468	0.510	0.539
40	0.110	0.207	0.264	0.313	0.368	0.405	0.439	0.479	0.507
45	0.103	0.194	0.248	0.294	0.347	0.382	0.414	0.453	0.479
50	0.097	0.184	0.235	0.279	0.329	0.363	0.393	0.430	0.456
55	0.093	0.175	0.224	0.266	0.314	0.346	0.375	0.411	0.435
60	0.089	0.168	0.214	0.255	0.300	0.331	0.360	0.394	0.418
65	0.085	0.161	0.206	0.244	0.289	0.318	0.346	0.379	0.402
70	0.082	0.155	0.198	0.235	0.278	0.307	0.333	0.365	0.388
75	0.079	0.150	0.191	0.227	0.269	0.297	0.322	0.353	0.375
80	0.076	0.145	0.185	0.220	0.260	0.287	0.312	0.342	0.363
85	0.074	0.140	0.180	0.213	0.252	0.279	0.303	0.332	0.353
90	0.072	0.136	0.174	0.207	0.245	0.271	0.294	0.323	0.343
95	0.070	0.133	0.170	0.202	0.239	0.264	0.287	0.314	0.334
100	0.068	0.129	0.165	0.197	0.233	0.257	0.279	0.307	0.326

*To find Spearman's correlation coefficient that is associated with a certain chance of making a type I error, find the column corresponding with that value of α at the top of table ($\alpha(2)$ indicates a two-tailed value and $\alpha(1)$ indicates a one-tailed value) and the row corresponding to the sample's size in the leftmost column. The value in the body of the table where that column and row intersect is the absolute value of Spearman's correlation coefficient that is expected to occur in α of the samples when Spearman's correlation coefficient is equal to zero in the population.

Table B.6 Critical values of the Mann-Whitney U statistic*

$\alpha(2)$ $\alpha(1)$		0.20 0.10	0.10 0.05	0.05 0.025	0.02 0.01	0.01 0.005	0.005 0.0025	0.002 0.001	0.001 0.0005
n_s	n_L								
1	1	—	—	—	—	—	—	—	—
	2	—	—	—	—	—	—	—	—
	3	—	—	—	—	—	—	—	—
	4	—	—	—	—	—	—	—	—
	5	—	—	—	—	—	—	—	—
	6	—	—	—	—	—	—	—	—
	7	—	—	—	—	—	—	—	—
	8	—	—	—	—	—	—	—	—
	9	9	—	—	—	—	—	—	—
	10	10	—	—	—	—	—	—	—
	12	12	—	—	—	—	—	—	—
	14	14	—	—	—	—	—	—	—
	16	16	—	—	—	—	—	—	—
	18	18	—	—	—	—	—	—	—
	20	19	20	—	—	—	—	—	—
	22	21	22	—	—	—	—	—	—
	24	23	24	—	—	—	—	—	—
	26	25	26	—	—	—	—	—	—
	28	27	28	—	—	—	—	—	—
	30	28	30	—	—	—	—	—	—
	32	30	32	—	—	—	—	—	—
	34	32	34	—	—	—	—	—	—
	36	34	36	—	—	—	—	—	—
	38	36	38	—	—	—	—	—	—
1	40	37	39	40	—	—	—	—	—
2	2	—	—	—	—	—	—	—	—
	3	6	—	—	—	—	—	—	—
	4	8	—	—	—	—	—	—	—
	5	9	10	—	—	—	—	—	—
	6	11	12	—	—	—	—	—	—
	7	10	14	—	—	—	—	—	—
	8	14	15	16	—	—	—	—	—
	9	16	17	18	—	—	—	—	—
	10	17	19	20	—	—	—	—	—
	12	20	22	23	—	—	—	—	—
	14	23	25	27	28	—	—	—	—
	16	27	29	31	32	—	—	—	—
	18	30	32	34	36	—	—	—	—
	20	33	36	38	39	40	—	—	—
	22	36	39	41	43	44	—	—	—
	24	39	42	45	47	48	—	—	—
	26	42	46	48	51	52	—	—	—
	28	45	49	52	54	55	56	—	—
	30	48	53	55	58	59	60	—	—
	32	51	56	59	62	63	64	—	—
	34	55	59	63	65	67	68	—	—
	36	58	63	66	69	71	72	—	—
	38	61	66	70	73	75	76	—	—
	40	64	69	73	77	78	79	—	—

*To find a Mann-Whitney U statistic that is associated with a certain chance of making a type I error, find the column corresponding with that value of α at the top of table ($\alpha(2)$ indicates a two-tailed value and $\alpha(1)$ indicates a one-tailed value) and the row corresponding to the sample's size in the leftmost column. The value in the body of the table where that column and row intersect is the value of the Mann-Whitney U statistic that is expected to occur in α of the samples when there is no association between the groups in the population.

Table B.6   *Continued*

$\alpha(2)$		0.20	0.10	0.05	0.02	0.01	0.005	0.002	0.001
$\alpha(1)$		0.10	0.05	0.025	0.01	0.005	0.0025	0.001	0.0005
n_S	n_L								
2	32	51	56	59	62	63	64	--	--
	34	55	59	63	65	67	68	--	--
	36	58	63	66	69	71	72	--	--
	38	61	66	70	73	75	76	--	--
	40	64	69	73	77	78	79	--	--
3	3	8	9	--	--	--	--	--	--
	4	11	12	--	--	--	--	--	--
	5	13	14	15	--	--	--	--	--
	6	15	16	17	--	--	--	--	--
	7	15	19	20	21	--	--	--	--
	8	19	21	22	24	--	--	--	--
	9	22	23	25	26	27	--	--	--
	10	24	26	27	29	30	--	--	--
	12	28	31	32	34	35	36	--	--
	14	32	35	37	40	41	42	--	--
	16	37	40	42	45	46	47	--	--
	18	41	45	47	50	52	53	54	--
	20	45	49	52	55	57	58	60	--
	22	50	54	57	60	62	64	65	66
	24	54	59	62	66	68	69	71	72
	26	58	63	67	71	73	75	77	78
	28	63	68	72	76	79	80	82	83
	30	67	73	77	81	84	86	88	89
	32	71	77	82	87	89	91	94	95
	34	76	82	87	92	95	97	99	101
	36	80	87	92	97	100	103	105	106
	38	84	91	97	102	105	108	111	112
3	40	89	96	102	107	111	114	116	118
4	4	13	15	16	--	--	--	--	--
	5	16	18	19	20	--	--	--	--
	6	19	21	22	23	24	--	--	--
	7	20	24	25	27	28	--	--	--
	8	25	27	28	30	31	32	--	--
	9	27	30	32	33	35	36	--	--
	10	30	33	35	37	38	39	40	--
	12	36	39	41	43	45	46	48	--
	14	41	45	47	50	52	53	55	56
	16	47	50	53	57	59	60	62	63
	18	52	56	60	63	66	67	69	71
	20	58	62	66	70	72	75	77	78
	22	63	68	72	77	79	82	84	85
	24	69	74	79	83	86	89	91	93
	26	74	80	85	90	93	96	98	100
	28	80	86	91	96	100	103	106	108
4	30	85	92	97	103	107	110	113	115

Table B.6 *Continued*

α(2)	0.20	0.10	0.05	0.02	0.01	0.005	0.002	0.001
α(1)	0.10	0.05	0.025	0.01	0.005	0.0025	0.001	0.0005

n_S	n_L								
4	32	91	98	104	110	114	117	120	122
	34	96	104	110	116	120	124	127	130
	36	102	110	116	123	127	131	135	137
	38	107	116	122	130	134	138	142	144
4	40	113	121	129	136	141	145	149	152
5	5	20	21	23	24	25	--	--	--
	6	23	25	27	28	29	30	--	--
	7	24	29	30	32	34	35	--	--
	8	30	32	34	36	38	39	40	--
	9	33	36	38	40	42	43	44	45
	10	37	39	42	44	46	47	49	50
	12	43	47	49	52	54	56	58	59
	14	50	54	57	60	63	64	67	68
	16	57	61	65	68	71	73	75	77
	18	63	68	72	76	79	81	84	86
	20	70	75	80	84	87	90	93	95
	22	77	82	97	92	96	98	102	104
	24	84	90	95	100	104	107	110	113
	26	90	97	102	108	112	115	119	121
	28	97	104	110	116	120	124	128	130
	30	104	111	117	124	128	132	136	139
	32	110	118	125	132	137	141	145	148
	34	117	125	132	140	145	149	154	157
	36	124	132	140	148	153	158	163	166
	38	130	140	147	156	161	166	171	175
5	40	137	147	155	164	169	174	180	184
6	6	27	29	31	33	34	35	--	--
	7	29	34	36	38	39	40	42	--
	8	35	38	40	42	44	45	47	48
	9	39	42	44	47	49	50	52	53
	10	43	46	49	52	54	55	57	58
	12	51	55	58	61	63	65	68	69
	14	59	63	67	71	73	75	78	79
	16	67	71	75	80	83	85	88	90
	18	74	80	84	89	92	95	98	100
	20	82	88	93	98	102	105	108	111
	22	90	96	102	108	111	115	119	121
	24	98	105	111	117	121	125	129	132
	26	106	113	119	126	131	134	139	142
	28	114	122	128	135	140	144	149	152
6	30	122	130	137	145	150	154	159	163

Table B.6 *Continued*

$\alpha(2)$ $\alpha(1)$		0.20 0.10	0.10 0.05	0.05 0.025	0.02 0.01	0.01 0.005	0.005 0.0025	0.002 0.001	0.001 0.0005
n_S	n_L								
6	32	129	138	146	154	159	164	169	173
	34	137	147	154	163	169	174	179	183
	36	145	155	163	172	178	184	190	194
	38	153	163	172	182	188	193	200	204
6	40	161	172	181	191	197	203	210	214
7	7	36	38	41	43	45	46	48	49
	8	40	43	46	49	50	52	54	55
	9	45	48	51	54	56	58	60	61
	10	49	53	56	59	61	63	65	67
	12	58	63	66	70	72	75	77	79
	14	67	72	76	81	83	86	89	91
	16	76	82	86	91	94	97	101	103
	18	85	91	96	102	105	108	112	115
	20	94	101	106	112	116	120	124	126
	22	103	110	116	123	127	131	135	138
	24	112	120	126	133	138	142	147	150
	26	121	129	136	144	149	153	158	162
	28	130	139	146	154	160	164	170	174
	30	139	149	156	165	170	176	181	185
	32	148	158	166	175	181	187	193	197
	34	157	168	176	186	192	198	204	209
	36	166	177	186	196	203	209	216	221
	38	175	187	196	207	214	220	227	232
7	40	184	196	206	217	225	231	239	244
8	8	45	49	51	55	57	58	60	62
	9	50	54	57	61	63	65	67	68
	10	56	60	63	67	69	71	74	75
	12	66	70	74	79	81	84	87	89
	14	76	81	86	90	94	96	100	102
	16	86	92	97	102	106	109	113	115
	18	96	103	108	114	118	122	126	129
	20	106	113	119	126	130	134	139	142
	22	117	124	131	138	142	147	152	155
	24	127	135	142	150	155	159	165	168
	26	137	146	153	161	167	172	177	181
	28	147	156	164	173	179	184	190	195
	30	157	167	175	185	191	197	203	208
	32	167	178	187	197	203	209	216	221
	34	177	188	198	208	215	222	229	234
	36	188	199	209	220	228	234	242	247
	38	198	210	220	232	240	247	255	260
8	40	208	221	231	244	252	259	268	273

Table B.6 *Continued*

$\alpha(2)$		0.20	0.10	0.05	0.02	0.01	0.005	0.002	0.001
$\alpha(1)$		0.10	0.05	0.025	0.01	0.005	0.0025	0.001	0.0005
n_S	n_L								
9	9	56	60	64	67	70	72	74	76
	10	62	66	70	74	77	79	82	83
	12	73	78	82	87	90	93	96	98
	14	85	90	95	100	104	107	111	113
	16	96	102	107	113	117	121	125	128
	18	107	114	120	126	131	135	139	142
	20	118	126	132	140	144	149	154	157
	22	130	138	145	153	158	162	168	172
	24	141	150	157	166	171	176	182	186
	26	152	162	170	179	185	190	196	201
	28	164	174	182	192	198	204	211	215
	30	175	185	194	205	212	218	225	230
	32	186	197	207	218	225	231	239	244
	34	197	209	219	231	238	245	253	259
	36	209	221	232	244	252	259	267	273
	38	220	233	244	257	265	273	282	288
9	40	231	245	257	270	279	286	296	302
10	10	68	73	77	81	84	87	90	92
	12	81	86	91	96	99	102	106	108
	14	93	99	104	110	114	117	121	124
	16	106	112	118	124	129	133	137	140
	18	118	125	132	139	143	148	153	156
	20	130	138	145	153	158	163	168	172
	22	143	152	159	167	173	178	184	188
	24	155	165	173	182	188	193	200	204
	26	168	178	186	196	202	208	215	220
	28	180	191	200	210	217	223	231	236
	30	192	204	213	224	232	238	246	252
	32	205	217	227	239	246	253	262	267
	34	217	230	241	253	261	268	277	283
	36	229	243	254	267	276	284	293	299
	38	242	256	268	281	290	299	308	315
10	40	254	269	281	296	305	314	324	331

Table B.7   Critical values of the chi-square distribution[*]

α(l)	0.50	0.25	0.10	0.05	0.025	0.01	0.005	0.001
df								
1	0.455	1.323	2.706	3.841	5.024	6.635	7.879	10.828
2	1.386	2.773	4.605	5.991	7.378	9.210	10.597	13.816
3	2.366	4.108	6.251	7.815	9.348	11.345	12.838	16.266
4	3.357	5.385	7.779	9.488	11.143	13.277	14.860	18.467
5	4.351	6.626	9.236	11.070	12.833	15.086	16.750	20.515
6	5.348	7.841	10.645	12.592	14.449	16.812	18.548	22.458
7	6.346	9.037	12.017	14.067	16.013	18.475	20.278	24.322
8	7.344	10.219	13.362	15.507	17.535	20.090	21.955	26.124
9	8.343	11.389	14.684	16.919	19.023	21.666	23.589	27.877
10	9.342	12.549	15.987	18.307	20.483	23.209	25.188	29.588
11	10.341	13.701	17.275	19.675	21.920	24.725	26.757	31.264
12	11.340	14.845	18.549	21.026	23.337	26.217	28.300	32.909
13	12.340	15.984	19.812	22.362	24.736	27.688	29.819	34.528
14	13.339	17.117	21.064	23.685	26.119	29.141	31.319	36.123
15	14.339	18.245	22.307	24.996	27.488	30.578	32.801	37.697
16	15.338	19.369	23.542	26.296	28.845	32.000	34.267	39.252
17	16.338	20.489	24.769	27.587	30.191	33.409	35.718	40.790
18	17.338	21.605	25.989	28.869	31.526	34.805	37.156	42.312
19	18.338	22.718	27.204	30.144	32.852	36.191	38.582	43.820
20	19.337	23.828	28.412	31.410	34.170	37.566	39.997	45.315
21	20.337	24.935	29.615	32.671	35.479	38.932	41.401	46.797
22	21.337	26.039	30.813	33.924	36.781	40.289	42.796	48.268
23	22.337	27.141	32.007	35.172	38.076	41.638	44.181	49.728
24	23.337	28.241	33.196	36.415	39.364	42.980	45.559	51.179
25	24.337	29.339	34.382	37.652	40.646	44.314	46.928	52.620
26	25.336	30.435	35.563	38.885	41.923	45.642	48.290	54.052
27	26.336	31.528	36.741	40.113	43.195	46.963	49.645	55.476
28	27.336	32.620	37.916	41.337	44.461	48.278	50.993	56.892
29	28.336	33.711	39.087	42.557	45.722	49.588	52.336	58.301
30	29.336	34.800	40.256	43.773	46.979	50.892	53.672	59.703
35	34.336	40.223	46.059	49.802	53.203	57.342	60.275	66.619
40	39.335	45.616	51.805	55.758	59.342	63.691	66.766	73.402
45	44.335	50.985	57.505	61.656	65.410	69.957	73.166	80.077
50	49.335	56.334	63.167	67.505	71.420	76.154	79.490	86.661
55	54.335	61.665	68.796	73.311	77.380	82.292	85.749	93.168
60	59.335	66.981	74.397	79.082	83.298	88.379	91.952	99.607
65	64.335	72.285	79.973	84.821	89.177	94.422	98.105	105.99
70	69.334	77.577	85.527	90.531	95.023	100.43	104.22	112.32
75	74.334	82.858	91.061	96.217	100.84	106.39	110.29	118.60
80	79.334	88.130	96.578	101.88	106.63	112.33	116.32	124.84
85	84.334	93.394	102.08	107.52	112.39	118.24	122.33	131.04
90	89.334	98.650	107.57	113.15	118.14	124.12	128.30	137.21
95	94.334	103.90	113.04	118.75	123.86	129.97	134.25	143.34
100	99.334	109.14	118.50	124.34	129.56	135.81	140.17	149.45

[*]To locate a chi-square value, find the degrees of freedom in the leftmost column and the appropriate α at the top of the table (only one-tailed α are appropriate in the chi-square distribution). The number in the body of the table where this row and column intersect is the value from the chi-square distribution with that number of degrees of freedom and that corresponds to an area equal to α in the upper tail.

Table B.8 Critical values of the q distribution[*]

				$\alpha(2) = 0.10$					
k	**2**	**3**	**4**	**5**	**6**	**7**	**8**	**9**	**10**
df									
1	8.929	13.44	16.36	18.49	20.15	21.51	22.64	23.62	24.48
2	4.130	5.733	6.773	7.538	8.139	8.633	9.049	9.409	9.725
3	3.328	4.467	5.199	5.738	6.162	6.511	6.806	7.062	7.287
4	3.015	3.976	4.586	5.035	5.388	5.679	5.926	6.139	6.327
5	2.850	3.717	4.264	4.664	4.979	5.238	5.458	5.648	5.816
6	2.748	3.559	4.065	4.435	4.726	4.966	5.168	5.344	5.499
7	2.680	3.451	3.931	4.280	4.555	4.780	4.972	5.137	5.283
8	2.630	3.374	3.843	4.169	4.431	4.646	4.829	4.987	5.126
9	2.592	3.316	3.761	4.084	4.337	4.545	4.721	4.873	5.007
10	2.563	3.270	3.704	4.018	4.264	4.465	4.636	4.783	4.913
11	2.540	3.234	3.658	3.965	4.205	4.401	4.568	4.711	4.838
12	2.521	3.204	3.621	3.922	4.156	4.349	4.511	4.652	4.776
13	2.505	3.179	3.589	3.885	4.116	4.305	4.464	4.602	4.724
14	2.491	3.158	3.563	3.854	4.081	4.267	4.424	4.560	4.680
15	2.479	3.140	3.540	3.828	4.052	4.235	4.390	4.524	4.641
16	2.469	3.124	3.520	3.804	4.026	4.207	4.360	4.492	4.608
17	2.460	3.110	3.503	3.784	4.004	4.183	4.334	4.464	4.579
18	2.452	3.098	3.488	3.767	30984	4.161	4.311	4.440	4.554
19	2.455	3.087	3.474	3.751	3.966	4.142	4.290	4.418	4.531
20	2.439	3.078	3.462	3.736	3.950	4.124	4.271	4.398	4.510
30	2.400	3.017	3.648	3.648	3.851	4.016	4.155	4.275	4.381
40	2.381	2.988	3.349	3.605	3.803	3.963	4.099	4.215	4.317
50	2.372	2.974	3.584	3.584	3.586	3.937	4.071	4.185	4.286
60	2.363	2.959	3.562	3.562	3.562	3.911	4.042	4.155	4.254
∞	2.326	2.902	3.478	3.478	3.478	3.808	4.931	4.037	4.129

k	**11**	**12**	**13**	**14**	**15**	**16**	**17**	**18**	**19**
df									
1	25.24	25.92	26.54	27.10	27.62	28.10	28.54	28.96	29.35
2	10.01	10.26	10.49	10.70	10.89	11.07	11.24	11.39	11.54
3	7.487	7.667	7.832	7.982	8.120	8.249	8.368	8.479	8.584
4	6.495	6.645	6.783	6.909	7.025	7.133	7.233	7.327	7.414
5	5.966	6.101	6.223	6.336	6.440	6.536	6.626	6.710	6.789
6	5.637	5.762	5.875	5.979	6.075	6.164	6.247	6.325	6.398
7	5.413	5.530	5.637	5.735	5.826	5.910	5.988	6.061	6.130
8	5.250	5.362	5.464	5.558	5.644	5.274	5.799	5.869	5.935
9	5.127	5.234	5.333	5.423	5.506	5.583	5.655	5.723	5.786
10	5.029	5.134	5.229	5.317	5.397	5.472	5.542	5.607	5.668
11	4.951	5.053	5.146	5.231	5.309	5.382	5.450	5.514	5.573
12	4.886	4.986	5.077	5.160	5.236	5.308	5.374	5.436	4.495
13	4.832	4.930	5.019	5.100	5.176	5.245	5.311	5.372	5.429
14	4.786	4.882	4.970	5.050	5.124	5.192	5.256	5.316	5.373
15	4.746	4.841	4.927	5.006	5.079	5.147	5.209	5.269	5.324
16	4.712	4.805	4.890	4.968	5.040	5.107	5.169	5.227	5.282
17	4.682	4.774	4.858	4.935	5.005	5.071	5.133	5.190	5.244
18	4.655	4.746	4.829	4.905	4.975	5.040	5.101	5.158	5.211
19	4.631	4.721	4.803	4.879	4.948	5.012	5.073	5.129	5.182
20	4.609	4.699	4.780	4.855	4.924	4.987	5.047	5.103	5.155
30	4.474	4.559	4.635	4.706	4.770	4.830	4.866	4.939	4.988
40	4.408	4.490	4.564	4.632	4.695	4.752	4.807	4.857	4.905
50	4.375	4.456	4.519	4.595	4.657	4.714	4.767	4.816	4.863
60	4.342	4.421	4.493	4.558	4.619	4.675	4.727	4.775	4.821
∞	4.211	4.285	4.351	4.412	4.468	4.519	4.568	4.612	4.654

[*]To find a value of q, first locate the table headed by the appropriate value of α. Then, find the degrees of freedom in the leftmost column and the number of means involved in the comparison (k) in the top row of the table. Where this row and column intersect is the value of q corresponding to an area of α in the q distribution with that number of degrees of freedom and k means.

Table B.8   *Continued*

$\alpha(2) = 0.05$								
k	2	3	4	5	6	7	8	9	10
df								
1	17.97	26.98	32.82	37.08	40.17	43.12	45.40	47.36	49.07
2	6.085	8.331	9.798	10.88	11.74	12.44	13.03	13.54	13.99
3	4.501	5.910	6.825	7.502	8.037	8.478	8.853	9.177	9.462
4	3.927	5.040	5.757	6.287	6.707	7.053	7.347	7.602	7.826
5	3.635	4.602	5.218	5.673	6.033	6.330	6.582	6.802	6.995
6	3.461	4.339	4.896	5.305	5.628	5.895	6.122	6.319	6.493
7	3.344	4.165	4.681	5.060	5.359	5.606	5.815	5.998	6.158
8	3.261	4.041	4.529	4.886	5.167	5.399	5.597	5.767	5.918
9	3.199	3.949	4.415	4.756	5.024	5.244	5.432	5.595	5.739
10	3.151	3.877	4.327	4.654	4.912	5.124	5.305	5.461	5.599
11	3.133	3.820	4.256	4.574	4.823	5.028	5.202	5.353	5.487
12	3.082	3.773	4.199	4.508	4.751	4.950	5.119	5.265	5.395
13	3.055	3.735	4.151	4.453	4.690	4.885	5.049	5.192	5.318
14	3.033	3.702	4.111	4.407	4.639	4.829	4.990	5.131	5.254
15	3.014	3.674	4.076	4.367	4.595	4.782	4.940	5.077	5.198
16	2.998	3.649	4.046	4.333	4.557	4.741	4.897	5.031	5.150
17	2.984	3.628	4.020	4.303	4.524	4.705	4.858	4.991	5.108
18	2.971	3.609	3.997	4.277	4.495	4.673	4.824	4.956	5.071
19	2.960	3.593	3.977	4.253	4.469	4.645	4.794	4.924	5.038
20	2.950	3.578	3.958	4.232	4.445	4.620	4.768	4.896	5.008
30	2.888	3.486	3.845	4.102	4.302	4.464	4.602	4.720	4.824
40	2.858	3.442	3.791	4.039	4.232	4.389	4.521	4.635	4.735
50	2.844	4.423	3.764	4.008	4.196	4.352	4.481	4.593	4.691
60	2.829	3.399	3.399	3.977	4.163	4.314	4.441	4.550	4.646
∞	2.772	3.314	3.633	3.858	4.030	4.170	4.286	4.387	4.474

k	11	12	13	14	15	16	17	18	19
df								
1	50.59	51.96	53.20	54.33	55.36	56.32	57.22	58.04	58.83
2	14.39	14.75	15.08	15.38	15.65	15.91	16.14	16.37	16.57
3	9.717	9.946	10.15	10.35	10.53	10.69	10.84	10.98	11.11
4	8.027	8.208	8.373	8.525	8.664	8.794	8.914	9.028	9.134
5	7.168	7.324	7.466	7.596	7.717	7.828	7.932	8.030	8.122
6	6.649	6.789	6.917	7.034	7.143	7.244	7.338	7.426	7.508
7	6.302	6.431	6.550	6.658	6.759	6.852	6.939	7.020	7.097
8	6.054	6.175	6.287	6.389	6.483	6.571	6.653	6.729	6.802
9	5.867	5.983	6.089	6.186	6.276	6.359	6.437	6.510	6.579
10	5.722	5.833	5.935	6.028	6.114	6.194	6.269	6.339	6.405
11	5.605	5.713	5.811	5.901	5.984	6.062	6.134	6.202	6.265
12	5.511	5.615	5.710	5.798	5.878	5.953	6.023	6.089	6.151
13	5.431	5.533	5.625	5.711	5.789	5.862	5.931	5.995	6.055
14	5.364	5.463	5.554	5.637	5.714	5.786	5.852	5.915	5.974
15	5.306	5.404	5.493	5.574	5.649	5.720	5.785	5.846	5.904
16	5.256	5.352	5.439	5.520	5.593	5.662	5.727	5.786	5.843
17	5.212	5.307	5.392	5.471	5.544	5.612	5.675	5.734	5.790
18	5.174	5.267	5.352	5.429	5.501	5.568	5.630	5.688	5.743
19	5.140	5.231	5.315	5.391	5.462	5.528	5.589	5.647	5.701
20	5.108	5.199	5.282	5.357	5.427	5.493	5.553	5.610	5.663
30	4.917	5.001	5.077	5.147	5.211	5.271	5.327	5.379	5.429
40	4.824	4.904	4.977	5.044	5.106	5.163	5.216	5.266	5.313
50	4.778	4.856	4.928	4.993	5.054	5.110	5.162	5.210	5.256
60	4.732	4.808	4.878	4.942	5.001	5.056	5.107	5.154	5.199
∞	4.552	4.622	4.685	4.743	4.796	4.845	4.891	4.934	4.974

Table B.8 *Continued*

$\alpha(2) = 0.01$									
k	2	3	4	5	6	7	8	9	10
df									
1	90.03	135.0	164.3	185.6	202.2	215.8	227.2	237.0	245.6
2	14.04	19.02	22.29	24.72	26.63	28.20	29.53	30.68	31.69
3	8.261	10.62	12.17	13.33	14.24	15.00	15.64	16.20	16.69
4	6.512	8.120	9.173	9.958	10.58	11.10	11.55	11.93	12.27
5	5.702	6.976	7.804	8.421	8.913	9.321	9.669	9.972	10.24
6	5.243	6.331	7.033	7.556	7.973	8.318	8.613	8.869	9.097
7	4.949	5.919	6.543	7.005	7.373	7.679	7.939	8.166	8.368
8	4.746	5.635	6.204	6.625	6.960	7.237	7.474	7.681	7.863
9	4.596	5.428	5.957	6.348	6.658	6.915	7.134	7.325	7.495
10	4.482	5.270	5.769	6.163	6.428	6.669	6.875	7.055	7.213
11	4.392	5.146	5.621	5.970	6.247	6.476	6.672	6.842	6.992
12	4.320	5.046	5.502	5.836	6.101	6.321	6.507	6.670	6.814
13	4.260	4.964	5.404	5.727	5.981	6.192	6.372	6.528	6.667
14	4.210	4.895	5.322	5.634	5.881	6.085	6.258	6.409	6.543
15	4.168	4.836	5.252	5.556	5.796	5.994	6.162	6.309	6.439
16	4.131	4.786	5.192	5.489	5.722	5.915	6.079	6.022	6.349
17	4.099	4.742	5.140	5.430	5.659	5.847	6.007	6.147	6.270
18	4.071	4.703	5.094	5.379	5.603	5.788	5.944	6.081	6.201
19	4.046	4.670	5.054	5.334	5.554	5.735	5.889	6.022	6.141
20	4.024	4.639	5.018	5.294	5.510	5.688	5.839	5.970	6.087
30	3.889	4.455	4.799	5.048	5.242	5.401	5.536	5.653	5.756
40	3.825	4.367	4.696	4.931	5.114	5.265	5.392	5.502	5.559
50	3.794	4.325	4.645	4.874	5.014	5.198	5.322	5.429	5.503
60	3.762	4.282	4.595	4.818	4.991	5.133	5.253	5.356	5.447
∞	3.643	4.120	4.403	4.603	4.757	4.882	4.987	5.078	5.157
k	11	12	13	14	15	16	17	18	19
df									
1	253.2	260.0	266.2	271.8	277.0	281.8	286.3	290.4	294.3
2	32.59	33.40	34.13	34.81	35.43	36.00	36.53	37.03	37.50
3	17.13	17.53	17.89	18.22	18.52	18.81	19.07	19.32	19.55
4	12.57	12.84	13.09	13.32	13.53	13.73	13.91	14.08	14.24
5	10.48	10.70	10.89	11.08	11.24	11.40	11.55	11.68	11.81
6	9.301	9.485	9.653	9.808	9.951	10.08	10.21	10.32	10.43
7	8.548	8.711	8.860	8.997	9.124	9.242	9.353	9.456	9.554
8	8.027	8.176	8.312	8.436	8.552	8.659	8.760	8.854	8.943
9	7.647	7.784	7.910	8.025	8.132	8.232	8.325	8.412	8.495
10	7.356	7.485	7.603	7.712	7.812	7.906	7.993	8.076	8.153
11	7.128	7.250	7.362	7.465	7.560	7.649	7.732	7.809	7.883
12	6.943	7.060	7.167	7.265	7.356	7.441	7.520	7.594	7.665
13	6.791	6.903	7.006	7.101	7.188	7.269	7.345	7.417	7.485
14	6.664	6.772	6.871	6.962	7.047	7.126	7.199	7.268	7.333
15	6.555	6.660	6.757	6.845	6.927	7.003	7.074	7.142	7.204
16	6.462	6.564	6.658	6.744	6.823	6.898	6.967	7.032	7.093
17	6.381	6.480	6.572	6.656	6.734	6.806	6.873	6.937	6.997
18	6.310	6.407	6.497	6.579	6.655	6.725	6.792	6.854	6.912
19	6.247	6.342	6.430	6.510	6.585	6.654	6.719	6.780	6.837
20	6.191	6.285	6.371	6.450	6.523	6.591	6.654	6.714	6.771
30	5.849	5.932	6.008	6.078	6.143	6.203	6.259	6.311	6.361
40	5.686	5.764	5.835	5.900	5.961	6.017	6.069	6.119	6.165
50	5.607	5.682	5.751	5.814	5.873	5.927	5.978	6.025	6.060
60	5.528	5.601	5.667	5.728	5.785	5.837	5.886	6.931	5.974
∞	5.227	5.290	5.348	5.400	5.448	5.493	5.535	5.611	5.611

Table B.8 *Continued*

					$\alpha(2) = 0.001$				
k	2	3	4	5	6	7	8	9	10
df									
1	900.3	1351.	1643.	1856.	2022.	2158.	2272.	2370.	2455.
2	44.69	60.42	70.77	78.43	84.49	89.46	93067	97.30	100.5
3	18.28	23.32	26.65	29.13	31.11	32.74	34.12	35.33	36.39
4	12.18	14.99	16.84	18.23	19.34	20.26	21.04	21.73	22.33
5	9.714	11.67	12.96	13.93	14.71	15.35	15.90	16.38	16.81
6	8.427	9.960	10.97	11.72	12.32	12.83	13.26	13.63	13.97
7	7.648	8.930	9.763	10.40	10.90	11.32	11.68	11.99	12.27
8	7.130	8.250	8.978	9.522	9.958	10.32	10.64	10.91	11.15
9	6.762	7.768	8.419	8.906	9.295	9.619	9.897	10.14	10.36
10	6.487	7.411	8.006	8.450	8.804	9.099	9.352	9.573	9.769
11	6.275	7.136	7.687	8.098	8.426	8.699	8.933	9.138	9.319
12	6.106	6.917	7.436	7.821	8.127	8.383	8.601	8.793	8.962
13	5.970	6.740	7.231	7.595	7.885	8.126	8.333	8.513	8.673
14	5.856	6.594	7.062	7.409	7.685	7.195	8.110	8.282	8.434
15	5.760	6.470	6.290	7.252	7.517	7.736	7.925	8.088	8.234
16	5.678	6.365	6.799	7.119	7.374	7.585	7.766	7.923	8.063
17	5.608	6.275	6.695	7.005	7.250	7.454	7.629	7.781	7.916
18	5.546	6.196	6.604	6.905	7.143	7.341	7.510	7.657	7.788
19	5.492	6.127	6.525	6.817	7.049	7.242	7.405	7.549	7.676
20	5.444	6.065	6.454	6.740	6.966	7.154	7.313	7.453	7.577
30	5.156	5.698	6.033	6.278	6.470	6.628	6.763	6.880	6.984
40	5.022	5.528	5.838	6.063	6.240	6.386	6.509	6.616	6.711
50	4.958	5.447	5.746	5.902	6.131	6.271	6.389	6.491	6.581
60	4.894	5.365	5.653	5.860	6.022	6.155	6.268	6.366	6.451
∞	4.654	5.063	5.309	5.619	5.619	5.730	5.823	5.093	5.973

k	11	12	13	14	15	16	17	18	19
df									
1	2532.	2600.	2662.	2718.	2770.	28.18	2863.	2904.	2943.
2	103.3	105.9	108.2	110.4	112.3	114.2	115.9	117.4	118.9
3	37.34	38.20	38.98	39.69	40.35	40.97	41.54	42.07	42.58
4	22.87	23.36	23.81	24.21	24.59	24.94	25.27	25.58	25.87
5	17.18	17.53	17.85	18.13	18.41	18.66	18.89	19.10	19.31
6	14.27	14.54	14.79	15.01	15.22	15.42	15.60	15.78	15.94
7	12.52	12.74	12.95	13.14	13.32	13.48	13.64	13.78	13.92
8	11.36	11.56	11.74	11.91	12.06	12.21	12.34	12.47	12.59
9	10.55	10.73	10.89	11.03	11.08	11.30	11.42	11.54	11.64
10	9.946	10.11	10.25	10.64	10.52	10.64	10.75	10.85	10.95
11	9.482	9.630	9.766	9.892	10.01	10.12	10.22	10.31	10.41
12	9.115	9.254	9.381	9.489	9.606	9.707	9.802	9.891	9.975
13	8.817	8.948	9.068	9.178	9.281	9.376	9.466	9.550	9.629
14	8.571	8.696	8.809	8.914	9.012	9.103	9.188	9.267	9.343
15	8.365	8.483	8.592	8.693	8.786	8.872	8.954	9.030	9.102
16	8.189	8.303	8.407	8.504	8.593	8.676	8.755	8.828	8.897
17	8.037	8.148	8.248	8.342	8.427	8.508	8.583	8.654	8.720
18	7.906	8.012	8.110	8.199	8.283	8.361	8.434	8.502	8.567
19	7.790	7.893	7.988	8.075	8.156	8.232	8.303	8.369	8.432
20	7.688	7.788	7.880	7.966	8.044	8.118	8.186	8.251	8.312
30	7.077	7.162	7.239	7.310	7.375	7.437	7.494	7.548	7.599
40	6.796	6.872	6.942	7.007	7.067	7.122	7.174	7.223	7.269
50	6.762	6.735	6.802	6.864	6.871	6.973	7.023	7.069	7.113
60	6.528	6.598	6.661	6.720	6.774	6.824	6.871	6.914	6.965
∞	6.036	6.092	6.144	6.191	6.234	6.274	6.312	6.347	6.380

Table B.9   Critical values of Kruskal-Wallis H statistics*

n_1	n_2	n_3	n_4	n_5	$\alpha(2)$ 0.10	0.05	0.02	0.01	0.005	0.002	0.001
2	2	2			4.571						
3	2	1			4.286						
3	2	2			4.500	4.714					
3	3	1			4.571	5.143					
3	3	2			4.556	5.361	6.250				
3	3	3			4.622	5.600	6.489	(7.200)	7.200		
4	2	1			4.500						
4	2	2			4.458	5.333	6.000				
4	3	1			4.056	5.208					
4	3	2			4.511	5.444	6.144	6.444	7.000		
4	3	3			4.709	5.791	6.564	6.745	7.318	8.018	
4	4	1			4.167	4.967	(6.667)	6.667			
4	4	2			4.555	5.455	6.600	7.036	7.282	7.855	
4	4	3			4.545	5.598	6.712	7.144	7.598	8.227	8.909
4	4	4			4.654	5.692	6.962	7.654	8.000	8.654	9.269
5	2	1			4.200	5.000					
5	2	2			4.373	5.160	6.000	6.533			
5	3	1			4.018	4.960	6.044				
5	3	2			4.651	5.251	6.124	6.909	7.182		
5	3	3			4.533	5.648	6.533	7.079	7.636	8.048	8.727
5	4	1			3.987	4.985	6.431	6.955	7.364		
5	4	2			4.541	5.273	6.505	7.205	7.573	8.114	8.591
5	4	3			4.549	5.656	6.676	7.445	7.927	8.481	8.795
5	4	4			4.619	5.657	6.953	7.760	8.189	8.868	9.168
5	5	1			4.109	5.127	6.145	7.309	8.182		
5	5	2			4.623	5.338	6.446	7.338	8.131	6.446	7.338
5	5	3			4.545	5.705	6.866	7.578	8.316	8.809	9.521
5	5	4			4.523	5.666	7.000	7.823	8.523	9.163	9.606
5	5	5			4.940	5.780	7.220	8.000	8.780	9.620	9.920
6	1	1			-----						
6	2	1			4.200	4.822					
6	2	2			4.545	5.345	6.182	6.982			
6	3	1			3.909	4.855	6.236				
6	3	2			4.682	5.348	6.227	6.970	7.515	8.182	
6	3	3			4.538	5.615	6.590	7.410	7.872	8.628	9.346
6	4	1			4.038	4.947	6.174	7.106	7.614		
6	4	2			4.494	5.340	6.571	7.340	7.846	8.494	8.827
6	4	3			4.604	5.610	6.725	7.500	8.033	8.918	9.170
6	4	4			4.595	5.681	6.900	7.795	8.381	9.167	9.861
6	5	1			4.128	4.990	6.138	7.182	8.077	8.515	

*To find a value of H, find the numbers of observations in each of the groups of dependent variable values in the leftmost column. It does not matter which group is considered group 1, etc.. Where this row and column intersect is the value of H that is expected to occur in α of the samples when there are differences between the groups in the population.

Table B.9 *Continued*

n_1	n_2	n_3	n_4	n_5	$\alpha(2)$ 0.10	0.05	0.02	0.01	0.005	0.002	0.001
6	5	2			4.596	5.338	6.585	7.376	8.196	8.967	9.189
6	5	3			4.535	5.602	6.829	7.590	8.314	9.150	9.669
6	5	4			4.522	5.661	7.018	7.936	8.643	9.458	9.960
6	5	5			4.547	5.729	7.110	8.028	8.859	9.771	10.271
6	6	1			4.000	4.945	6.286	7.121	8.165	9.077	9.692
6	6	2			4.438	5.410	6.667	7.467	8.210	9.219	9.752
6	6	3			4.558	5.625	6.900	7.725	8.458	9.458	10.150
6	6	4			4.548	5.724	7.107	8.000	8.754	9.662	10.342
6	6	5			4.542	5.765	7.152	8.124	8.987	9.948	10.524
6	6	6			4.643	5.801	7.240	8.222	9.170	10.187	10.889
7	7	7			4.594	5.819	7.332	8.378	9.373	10.516	11.310
8	8	8			4.595	5.805	7.355	8.465	9.495	10.805	11.705
2	2	1	1		-----						
2	2	2	1		5.357	5.679					
2	2	2	2		5.667	6.167	(6.667)	6.667			
3	1	1	1		-----						
3	2	1	1		5.143						
3	2	2	1		5.556	5.833	6.500				
3	2	2	2		5.644	6.333	6.978	7.133	7.533		
3	3	1	1		5.333	6.333					
3	3	2	1		5.689	6.244	6.689	7.200	7.400		
3	3	2	2		5.745	6.527	7.182	7.636	7.873	8.018	8.455
3	3	3	1		5.655	6.600	7.109	7.400	8.055	8.345	
3	3	3	2		5.879	6.727	7.636	8.105	8.379	8.803	9.030
3	3	3	3		6.026	7.000	7.872	8.538	8.897	9.462	9.513
4	1	1	1		-----						
4	2	1	1		5.250	5.833					
4	2	2	1		5.533	6.133	6.667	7.000			
4	2	2	2		5.755	6.545	7.091	7.391	7.964	8.291	
4	3	1	1		5.067	6.178	6.711	7.067			
4	3	2	1		5.591	6.309	7.018	7.455	7.773	8.182	
4	3	2	2		5.750	6.621	7.530	7.871	8.273	8.689	8.909
4	3	3	1		5.689	6.545	7.485	7.758	8.212	8.697	9.182
4	3	3	2		5.872	6.795	7.763	8.333	8.718	9.167	8.455
4	3	3	3		6.016	6.984	7.995	8.659	9.253	9.709	10.016
4	4	1	1		5.182	5.945	7.091	7.909	7.909		
4	4	2	1		5.568	6.386	7.364	7.886	8.341	8.591	8.909
4	4	2	2		5.808	6.731	7.750	8.346	8.692	9.269	9.462
4	4	3	1		5.692	6.635	7.660	8.231	8.583	9.038	9.327
4	4	3	2		5.901	6.874	7.951	8.621	9.165	9.615	9.945

Table B.9 *Continued*

n_1	n_2	n_3	n_4	n_5	$\alpha(2)$ 0.10	0.05	0.02	0.01	0.005	0.002	0.001
4	4	3	3		6.019	7.038	8.181	8.876	9.495	10.105	10.467
4	4	4	1		5.564	6.725	7.879	8.588	9.000	9.478	9.758
4	4	4	2		5.914	6.957	8.157	8.871	9.486	10.043	10.429
4	4	4	3		6.042	7.142	8.350	9.075	9.742	10.542	10.929
4	4	4	4		6.088	7.235	8.515	9.287	9.971	10.809	11.338
2	1	1	1	1	-----						
2	2	1	1	1	5.786						
2	2	2	1	1	6.250	6.750					
2	2	2	2	1	6.600	7.133	(7.533)	7.533			
2	2	2	2	2	6.982	7.418	8.073	8.291	(8.727)	8.727	
3	1	1	1	1	-----						
3	2	1	1	1	6.139	6.583					
3	2	2	1	1	6.511	6.800	7.400	7.600			
3	2	2	2	1	6.709	7.309	7.836	8.127	8.327	8.618	
3	2	2	2	2	6.955	7.682	8.303	8.682	8.985	9.273	9.364
3	3	1	1	1	6.311	7.111	7.467				
3	3	2	1	1	6.600	7.200	7.892	8.073	8.345		
3	3	2	2	1	6.788	7.591	8.258	8.576	8.924	9.167	9.303
3	3	2	2	2	7.026	7.910	8.667	9.115	9.474	9.769	10.026
3	3	3	1	1	6.788	7.576	8.242	8.424	8.848	(9.455)	9.455
3	3	3	2	1	6.910	7.769	8.590	9.051	9.410	9.769	9.974
3	3	3	2	2	7.121	8.044	9.011	9.505	9.890	10.330	10.637
3	3	3	3	1	7.077	8.000	8.879	9.451	9.846	10.286	10.549
3	3	3	3	2	7.210	8.200	9.267	9.876	10.333	10.838	11.171
3	3	3	3	3	7.333	8.333	9.467	10.200	10.733	10.267	11.667

Table B.10   Critical values of Dunn's Q statistics[*]

$\alpha(?)$	0.50	0.20	0.10	0.05	0.02	0.01	0.005	0.002	0.001
k									
2	0.674	1.282	1.645	1.960	2.327	2.576	2.807	3.091	3.291
3	1.383	1.834	2.128	2.394	2.713	2.936	3.144	3.403	3.588
4	1.732	2.128	2.394	2.639	2.936	3.144	3.342	3.588	3.765
5	1.960	2.327	2.576	2.807	3.091	3.291	3.481	3.719	3.891
6	2.128	2.475	2.713	2.936	3.209	3.403	3.588	3.820	3.988
7	2.261	2.593	2.823	3.038	3.304	3.494	3.675	3.902	4.067
8	2.369	2.690	2.914	3.124	3.384	3.570	3.748	3.972	4.134
9	2.461	2.773	2.992	3.197	3.453	3.635	3.810	4.031	4.191
10	2.540	2.845	3.059	3.261	3.512	3.692	3.865	4.083	4.241
11	2.609	2.908	3.119	3.317	3.565	3.743	3.914	4.129	4.286
12	2.671	2.965	3.172	3.368	3.613	3.789	3.957	4.171	4.326
13	2.726	3.016	3.220	3.414	3.656	3.830	3.997	4.209	4.363
14	2.777	3.062	3.264	3.456	3.695	3.868	4.034	4.244	4.397
15	2.823	3.105	3.304	3.494	3.731	3.902	4.067	4.276	4.428
16	2.866	3.144	3.342	3.529	3.765	3.935	4.098	4.305	4.456
17	2.905	3.181	3.376	3.562	3.796	3.965	4.127	4.333	4.483
18	2.942	3.215	3.409	3.593	3.825	3.993	4.154	4.359	4.508
19	2.976	3.246	3.439	3.622	3.852	4.019	4.179	4.383	4.532
20	3.008	3.276	3.467	3.649	3.878	4.044	4.203	4.406	4.554
21	3.038	3.304	3.494	3.675	3.902	4.067	4.226	4.428	4.575
22	3.067	3.331	3.519	3.699	3.925	4.089	4.247	4.448	4.595
23	3.094	3.356	3.543	3.722	3.947	4.110	4.268	4.468	4.614
24	3.120	3.380	3.566	3.744	3.968	4.130	4.287	4.486	4.632
25	3.144	3.403	3.588	3.765	3.988	4.149	4.305	4.504	4.649

[*]To find a value of Q, find the number of means of ranks in the comparison interval in the leftmost column, then locate the desired α value in the top row of the table. Where this column and row intersect is the value of Q that is expected to occur in α of the samples from a population in which there is no association between the groups.

Table B.11   **Ranks associated with the limits of a confidence interval for the median.**[*]

	90% Interval		95% Interval		99% Interval	
n	Lower	Upper	Lower	Upper	Lower	Upper
7	1	7	-	-	-	-
8	1	8	1	8	-	-
9	2	8	1	9	-	-
10	2	9	1	10	-	-
11	2	10	2	10	1	11
12	3	10	2	11	1	12
13	3	11	2	12	1	13
14	3	12	3	12	2	13
15	4	12	3	13	2	14
16	4	13	4	13	2	15
17	5	13	4	14	3	15
18	5	14	4	15	3	16
19	5	15	5	15	3	17
20	6	15	5	16	4	17
21	6	16	6	16	4	18
22	7	16	6	17	4	19
23	7	17	6	18	5	19
24	7	18	7	18	5	20
25	8	18	7	19	6	20
26	8	19	8	19	6	21
27	9	19	8	20	6	22
28	9	20	8	21	7	22
29	10	20	9	21	7	23
30	10	21	9	22	7	24
31	10	22	10	22	8	24
32	11	22	10	23	8	25
33	11	23	10	24	9	25
34	12	23	11	24	9	26
35	12	24	11	25	9	27
36	13	24	12	25	10	27
37	13	25	12	26	10	28
38	13	26	12	27	11	28
39	14	26	13	27	11	29
40	14	27	13	28	11	30

[*]To determine a confidence interval for a median, rank the data according to numeric magnitude. Then, locate the sample's size in the left-most column and the level of confidence in the top row. Where those two intersect, you will find the ranks of the data that correspond to the lower and upper limits of the confidence interval.

APPENDIX C

ANSWERS TO ODD EXERCISES

Chapter 1
1.1 D
1.3 B
1.5 D
1.7 E

Chapter 2
2.1 B
2.3 D
2.5 C

Chapter 3
3.1 D
3.3 C
3.5 E
3.7 D
3.9 C

Chapter 4
4.1 B
4.3 E
4.5 A
4.7 C

Chapter 5
5.1 E
5.3 B

Chapter 6
6.1 D
6.3 B
6.5 C
6.7 C
6.9 D

Chapter 7
7.1 E
7.3 E
7.5 C
7.7 D
7.9 B
7.11 E
7.13 A

Chapter 8
8.1 E
8.3 D
8.5 C

Chapter 9
9.1 A
9.3 E
9.5 C
9.7 D
9.9 C

Workbook to Accompany Introduction to Biostatistical Applications in Health Research with Microsoft® Office Excel®, First Edition. Robert P. Hirsch.
© 2016 John Wiley & Sons, Inc. Published 2016 by John Wiley & Sons, Inc.

Chapter 10

10.1 C
10.3 C
10.5 E
10.7 A
10.9 C
10.11 E
10.13 E
10.15 C
10.17 E
10.19 B

Chapter 11

11.1 E
11.3 C
11.5 E

Chapter 12

12.1 C
12.3 A,B
12.5 C
12.7 B
12.9 E
12.11 B
12.13 A
12.15 C

Chapter 13

13.1 C
13.3 A
13.5 C
13.7 E
13.9 D
13.11 B
13.13 D
13.15 E

Index

Workbook to Accompany Introduction to Biostatistical Applications in Health Research with Microsoft® Office Excel®, First Edition. Robert P. Hirsch.
© 2016 John Wiley & Sons, Inc. Published 2016 by John Wiley & Sons, Inc.

Printed and bound by CPI Group (UK) Ltd, Croydon, CR0 4YY

27/10/2024

14580476-0001